JN330435

東大醫學――蘭方医学からドイツ近代医学へ

The Dawn of Modern Medicine in Japan
From Dutch Medicine to German Medical Science

The University Museum, The University of Tokyo

2014

東大醫學――蘭方医学からドイツ近代医学へ

東京大学総合研究博物館

二〇一四年

Exhibition Organization Committee (in alphabetical order)

Yasunobu Hirata / Director, Tokyo Teishin Hospital
Masahisa Kaneko / Medical Museum, Graduate School of Medicine and Faculty of Medicine, The University of Tokyo
Toshimasa Kikuchi / Affiliate Assistant Professor, Intermediatheque Department, UMUT
Hajime Matsubara / Affiliate Assistant Professor, Intermediatheque Department, UMUT
Fumio Matsumoto / Affiliate Associate Professor, Museum Technology Department, UMUT
Kohei Miyazono / Dean and Professor, Graduate School of Medicine and Faculty of Medicine, The University of Tokyo
Ryozo Nagai / President, Jichi Medical University & President, Japanese Circulation Society & Professor emeritus, The University of Tokyo
Hiroto Nakatsubo / Affiliate Researcher, Intermediatheque Department, UMUT
Yoshiaki Nishino / Director, UMUT & Director, Intermediatheque
Kazuhiko Oe / Director, Museum of Health and Medicine & Professor, Graduate School of Medicine, The University of Tokyo
Shigeo Okabe / Professor, Graduate School of Medicine, The University of Tokyo
Kei Osawa / Affiliate Researcher, Intermediatheque Department, UMUT
Satoshi Sasaki / Professor, Graduate School of Medicine and Faculty of Medicine, The University of Tokyo
Hiroyuki Sekioka / Affiliate Associate Professor, Intermediatheque Department, UMUT
Ai Shiraishi / Affiliate Assistant Professor, Museum Technology Department, UMUT
Ayumi Terada / Affiliate Assistant Professor, Intermediatheque Department, UMUT
Eriko Ueno / Affiliate Researcher, Intermediatheque Department, UMUT

The present publication is the catalogue of the special exhibition *The Dawn of Modern Medicine in Japan: From Dutch Medicine to German Medical Science*, held within the special exhibition space of the JP Tower Museum Intermediatheque from March 19 to May 11, 2014. The exhibition is organized by the University Museum, the University of Tokyo (UMUT) with the cooperation of the Graduate School of Medicine of the University of Tokyo, the Japanese Circulation Society and the Museum of Health and Medicine depending on the Faculty of Medicine of the University of Tokyo and on the University of Tokyo Hospital. The edition of the catalogue and the conception of the exhibition are carried out by the Exhibition Organization Committee.

Notes on the Edition
- Key information is described in the following order: name of the specimen / date / area of production / producer / material / size / former collection / collection.
- Size indications are in millimeters.
- Descriptions are written by Yoshiaki Nishino and Koji Takayama of the University Museum, the University of Tokyo (UMUT), and by Masahisa Kaneko of the Medical Museum of the Graduate School of Medicine and Faculty of Medicine. English translation is supervised by Kei Osawa of the University Museum, the University of Tokyo (UMUT).

Photography
Pages 14-15, 20-23, 26-29, 36-39, 40-51: © Norihiro Ueno
All other pages: © The University Museum, The University of Tokyo (UMUT)

『東大醫學──蘭方医学からドイツ近代医学へ』展実行委員会（五十音順）

上野恵理子　東京大学総合研究博物館インターメディアテク研究部門特任研究員
大江和彦　　東京大学医学部・医学部附属病院「健康と医学の博物館」館長／東京大学大学院医学系研究科教授
大澤　啓　　東京大学総合研究博物館インターメディアテク研究部門特任研究員
岡部繁男　　東京大学大学院医学系研究科教授
金子仁久　　東京大学大学院医学系研究科・医学部標本室
菊池敏正　　東京大学総合研究博物館インターメディアテク研究部門特任助教
佐々木敏　　東京大学大学院医学系研究科教授
白石　愛　　東京大学総合研究博物館ミュージアム・テクノロジー研究部門特任助教
関岡裕之　　東京大学総合研究博物館インターメディアテク研究部門特任准教授
寺田鮎美　　東京大学総合研究博物館インターメディアテク研究部門特任助教
永井良三　　自治医科大学学長／日本循環器学会代表理事／東京大学名誉教授
中坪啓人　　東京大学総合研究博物館インターメディアテク研究部門特任研究員
西野嘉章　　東京大学総合研究博物館館長／インターメディアテク館長
平田恭信　　東京逓信病院院長
松原　始　　東京大学総合研究博物館インターメディアテク研究部門特任助教
松本文夫　　東京大学総合研究博物館ミュージアム・テクノロジー研究部門特任准教授
宮園浩平　　東京大学大学院医学系研究科・医学部教授／医学系研究科長・医学部長

　本書は2014年3月19日から5月11日にかけ、JPタワー「インターメディアテク」内の企画展示室において開催された特別展示『東大醫學──蘭方医学からドイツ近代医学へ』の図録である。上記の展覧会は東京大学総合研究博物館の主催、東京大学大学院医学系研究科、日本循環器学会および東京大学医学部・医学部附属病院「健康と医学の博物館」の協力になる特別展示であり、図録監修、展示構成は同展実行委員会がそれをおこなった。

凡例
－記載は、標本名および年代／産地／制作者／素材／サイズ／旧蔵／所蔵の順とした。
－サイズの単位はミリメートルとした。
－解説は東京大学総合研究博物館の西野嘉章、高山浩司、大学院医学系研究科・医学部標本室金子仁久が執筆した。英語監修は総合研究博物館の大澤啓が担当した。

写真
14-15, 20-23, 26-29, 36-39, 40-51頁：©上野則宏
上記以外：©東京大学総合研究博物館

Foreword

The University Museum, the University of Tokyo, with the collaboration of the Graduate School of Medicine and Faculty of Medicine, is organizing the special exhibition *The Dawn of Modern Medicine in Japan: From Dutch Medicine to German Medical Science*, in the special exhibition space "First Sight" of the Intermediatheque, located within the JP Tower on the Marunouchi side of Tokyo Station.

The medical specimens conserved both by the Medical Museum of the Graduate School of Medicine and Faculty of Medicine and by the Medicine Section of the Research Materials Department of the University Museum were in part shown in the context of the special exhibition *The Archaeology of Science*, held in autumn 1997 at the Yasuda Auditorium to commemorate the 120th anniversary of the University of Tokyo. However, by completing this corpus with the Miyake family collection issued from the illustrious family of doctors and conserved by the Research Department of the University Museum, the present exhibition publicizes for the first time in its entirety the heritage of modern Japanese medicine in its nascent stage.

The present exhibition is held in conjunction with the 78th Annual Scientific Meeting of the Japanese Circulation Society, and provides a unique opportunity to present the traces of the birth of modern medicine in Japan, not only to medical researchers in and outside Japan, but also to the general public.

In carrying out the present exhibition, we benefited from the cooperation and assistance of our partners from the Graduate School of Medicine and Faculty of Medicine, the Japanese Circulation Society as well as from the Museum of Health and Medicine depending on the Faculty of Medicine of the University of Tokyo and on the University of Tokyo Hospital. Our deep gratitude goes to each of them.

The Organizers
March, 2014

はじめに

　このたび東京大学総合研究博物館は、大学院医学系研究科・医学部のご協力を賜り、東京駅丸の内側ＪＰタワー「インターメディアテク」内の企画展スペース「FIRST SIGHT（ギャラリー1）」において、特別展示『東大醫學──蘭方医学からドイツ近代医学へ』を開催する運びとなりました。

　大学院医学系研究科・医学部標本室、総合研究博物館資料部医学部門に分蔵されている医学系学術標本は、平成9（1997）年秋に東京大学創立120周年を記念して安田講堂で開催された特別展示「学問のアルケオロジー」で、その一部を公開したこともありますが、総合研究博物館研究部に収蔵されている「近代医家三宅一族コレクション」と併せ、近代医学黎明期遺産としてまとめて一般公開が実現するのは、今回が初めてのこととなります。

　本展は、第78回日本循環器学会学術集会の東京開催に合わせて開催されるものであり、国内外の医学系研究者のみならず広く一般の方々にも日本近代医学誕生の軌跡をご覧頂く、絶好の機会になるものと思います。

　本展の実現にあたっては、東京大学大学院医学系研究科・医学部、日本循環器学会、東京大学医学部・医学部附属病院「健康と医学の博物館」の関係各位から、多大なご協力、ご支援を賜りました。最後になりましたが、関係者の方々に改めて御礼を申し上げる次第です。

主催者
2014年3月

Greetings

Medicine at the University of Tokyo as a Witness of Japanese Modernization

The commencement of the special exhibition *The Dawn of Modern Medicine in Japan: From Dutch Medicine to German Medical Science* will coincide with the 78th Annual Scientific Meeting of the Japanese Circulation Society.

Thanks to the generosity and efforts of Professors Yoshiaki Nishino (Director of the Intermediatheque), Kohei Miyazono (Dean of the Faculty of Medicine, the University of Tokyo) and Shigeo Okabe (Chief of the Historical Medical Data Room of the Faculty of Medicine, the University of Tokyo), this magnificent exhibition has been made possible.

The Faculty of Medicine of the University of Tokyo originated in 1858 when 83 Dutch-style medical doctors in Edo (present Tokyo) donated to establish a vaccination center. Several members of the center were employed as attending physicians of the shogun. In 1861, the vaccination center became the Medical Institute of the shogunate and was supported by the government.

After the Meiji Restoration, the Medical Institute of the shogunate was transformed into the Medical School of the Imperial University of Tokyo by inviting German professors, and was heavily supported by the Meiji government. Modernization of the nation needed a modern government, administrative offices and military forces, in all of which the Faculty of Medicine of the University of Tokyo was deeply involved. The collection of historical medical materials by the Faculty of Medicine of the University of Tokyo is valuable for not only Japanese researchers but also for researchers from abroad.

Medicine covers an extremely broad field. Therefore, it is by no means easy for any physician to understand its entirety. However, we can learn through the accomplishments of our forefathers. Therefore, this exhibition would seem to be an excellent opportunity for everybody.

I would like to express my sincerest gratitude to the University Museum, the University of Tokyo, which organized this exhibition, and to those who have contributed in order to make this important event possible.

Ryozo Nagai, M.D., Ph.D.
President, Jichi Medical University / President, Japanese Circulation Society / Professor emeritus, The University of Tokyo

ごあいさつ

日本の近代化の目撃者としての東大医学

　医学史展示『東大醫學──蘭方医学からドイツ近代医学へ』の開催にあたり、ご挨拶を申し上げます。今回の展覧会は、東京国際フォーラムにおける第78回日本循環器学会学術集会の開催にあわせて、東京大学が収集してきた幕末から明治期にかけての近代医学の資料を、学会参加者や市民に公開できればと考え、西野嘉章東京大学総合研究博物館長、宮園浩平東京大学医学部長、岡部繁男東京大学解剖学教授にご相談したところから、企画が始まりました。

　東京大学医学部は、1858年に江戸の蘭方医たちが設立した種痘所を前身とし、すでに150年を超える歴史があります。明治維新以前は幕府の西洋医学所であり、明治以後は日本最初の近代的な医学校として政府の手厚い保護を受けてきました。近代国家には近代的な行政府や軍とともに、近代医学が必須です。このため東京大学医学部は日本の近代化の過程と密接な関係にあり、医学部資料室には日本における近代医学の受容、とくに蘭学からドイツ医学への転換を示す貴重な資料が多数残されています。なかには欧米で失われた資料もあり、国内だけでなく海外の研究者の関心を呼ぶと期待しております。

　医学は膨大な領域を対象としており、その全貌を把握することは容易でありません。先人の苦闘の歴史を辿ることによって、本来の医学が何をめざすべきか示唆を得ることができます。『東大醫學──蘭方医学からドイツ近代医学へ』はわが国の近代医学の源流を探る絶好の機会となりました。医学と医療に関心のある多くの人々にご覧いただきたいと思います。

　最後に、主催者の東京大学総合研究博物館および本企画にご協力いただいた東京大学の関係者に心より御礼を申し上げます。

永井良三
自治医科大学学長／日本循環器学会代表理事／東京大学名誉教授

Greetings

The Evolution of Modern Medicine in Japan

The collection of medical specimens accumulated by the University of Tokyo is outstanding, both in quantity and in nature. It is no exaggeration to state that it is a first-rate corpus, bearing comparison with any collection held by important medical institutions throughout the world. This is quite natural. Since its establishment in 1877, the Faculty of Medicine of the University of Tokyo concentrated talented persons, and it benefited from research funds largely surpassing that of other institutions. However, the collection and the maintenance of medical specimens are far from being easy. We have to think of all the effort and passion devoted by our predecessors in managing this collection, overcoming numerous difficulties starting with the Great Kanto Earthquake and through the wartime ravages and evacuation up to student protests, in order to constitute the extant collection, unique in Japan.

Although they are generically referred to as "medical specimens," the exhibited items are diverse in content. They are not limited to body specimens. In effect, there are numerous materials used for education and research, such as manmade models, medical instruments and laboratory equipment. With the advent of an era calling out for the respect of private information and human rights, the public exhibition of body specimens encounters difficulties, at least within Japan. As a side effect, the opportunity to present related historical documentation such as models and instruments becomes rare, leading historical research on medicine to the path of decline.

The aim of the present exhibition is to present in a reconstituted form the evolution of modern medical science in Japan, through the medical heritage dating from the end of the shogunate to the first half of the Meiji period. This constitutes the first opportunity for the University Museum to exhibit in their totality to the general public these precious historical documents pertaining to medicine. To each member of the Graduate School of Medicine and Faculty of Medicine who acceded to our earnest wish to organize an exhibition of medical specimens, and who supported us in realizing it, I would like to take this opportunity to express all my gratitude.

Yoshiaki Nishino
Director, The University Museum, The University of Tokyo / Intermediatheque

ごあいさつ

日本における近代医学の歩み

　東京大学に蓄積されている医学標本コレクションは、その量と質の両面において突出している。世界の有力な医学研究機関の有するコレクションのどれと比べても遜色のない、第一級の資料体といって過言ではない。それも当然である。明治10(1877)年の創学以来、東京大学の医学部には優秀な人材が集中し、他機関にまさる研究費が投入されてきたからである。しかし、医学標本の収集蓄積と維持管理は容易でない。関東大震災をはじめ、戦禍疎開や大学紛争など、数多の困難を乗り越え、国内随一のコレクションとして「現在」するまでに、管理にあたる先達たちがどれほどの労力と情熱を傾けてきたか、そのことに思いを致さねばならない所以である。

　ひとくちに医学標本といっても、内容は様々である。生体標本だけではない。人造模型や医療器具・実験用具など、教育や研究に供されてきた数多の資料があるからである。個人情報や人権尊重が叫ばれる時代となり、少なくとも国内では生体標本の一般公開が困難を来している。それに曳きずられ、模型や器具といった周辺史料を公開する機会も減っており、結果として医学史研究は衰退の一途を辿っている。

　本展の狙いは、日本における近代医学の歩みを、幕末から明治前半の医学遺産をもって再構成して見せることにある。貴重な医学史資料をまとめて公開するのは、総合研究博物館にとって初めての機会である。医学標本展示を実現したいというわれわれの切なる願いをくみ取り、展示の実現に御協力くださった大学院医学系研究科・医学部の関係各位に、この場をかりて心より御礼を申し上げたい。

西野嘉章
東京大学総合研究博物館館長／インターメディアテク館長

Catalogue of Exhibited Items

The Collection of the Graduate School of Medicine and Faculty of Medicine

At the University of Tokyo, the Medical Museum of the Graduate School of Medicine and Faculty of Medicine is the best equipped facility in terms of management and exhibition of specimens. The medical specimens collected by the University of Tokyo since its establishment in 1877 are manifold, including among others fundamental specimen collections for education and research pertaining to the anatomy and physiology of the human body, as well as specimens of defined pathologies and symptoms. At the same time, the total quantity of such specimens has considerably increased. Among this colossal collection, and in spite of the limited quantity of concerned specimens, the heritage of the dawn of modern medicine should be noted for its historical significance. From the end of the shogunate to the Meiji period, Japan has introduced modern medicine from the West. The first step toward such a movement was the education of persons who were to carry out Western medicine. Western-style education was thus implemented under the guidance of foreign government advisors. Next, outstanding young researchers were sent abroad to study modern medicine on site. However, during this period, along with the collapse of the Tokugawa shogunate and the establishment of the Meiji government, the Japanese medical world experienced the fundamental conversion from Dutch-style medicine to German-style medicine. It was not until the Ordinance on Imperial Universities and the institutional reorganization into the Tokyo Imperial University, that Japanese medical researchers having studied in the West were able to publicize the results of their personal research on an international scale.

展示品解説

医学系研究科・医学部コレクション

　東京大学大学院医学系研究科・医学部標本室は、大学のなかでもっとも整備の行き届いた標本管理・公開施設である。明治10(1877)年の創学以来、東京大学が収集・蓄積してきた医学系学術標本は、人体構造や生理システムに関する基礎的な教育研究標本のコレクション、特異な病理標本や症例標本のコレクションなど、多岐にわたると同時にその全体量も膨大なものに膨れ上がっている。その膨大な標本コレクションのなかで、数は少ないにしても、歴史的な重要性において特筆すべきは、近代医学の黎明期の遺産である。幕末から明治にかけ、日本は西洋から近代医学を導入している。その第一歩は西洋医学を担う人材の育成であった。まずは御雇い外国人教師の招聘に始まる西洋式教育の実践。つぎは優秀な若手人材を海外に派遣し、現地で近代医学を修める欧米留学の推進。しかし、そうする間にも、徳川幕府の崩壊、明治政府の樹立と推移するなかで、オランダ式医学からドイツ式医学への大転換を経験したのが、日本の医学界だったのである。欧米に学んだ日本人医学者が、帰国後、独自の研究を基に国際的な研究業績を公表できるようになるのは、帝国大学令をもって東京帝国大学へ改組されてからのことになる。

014

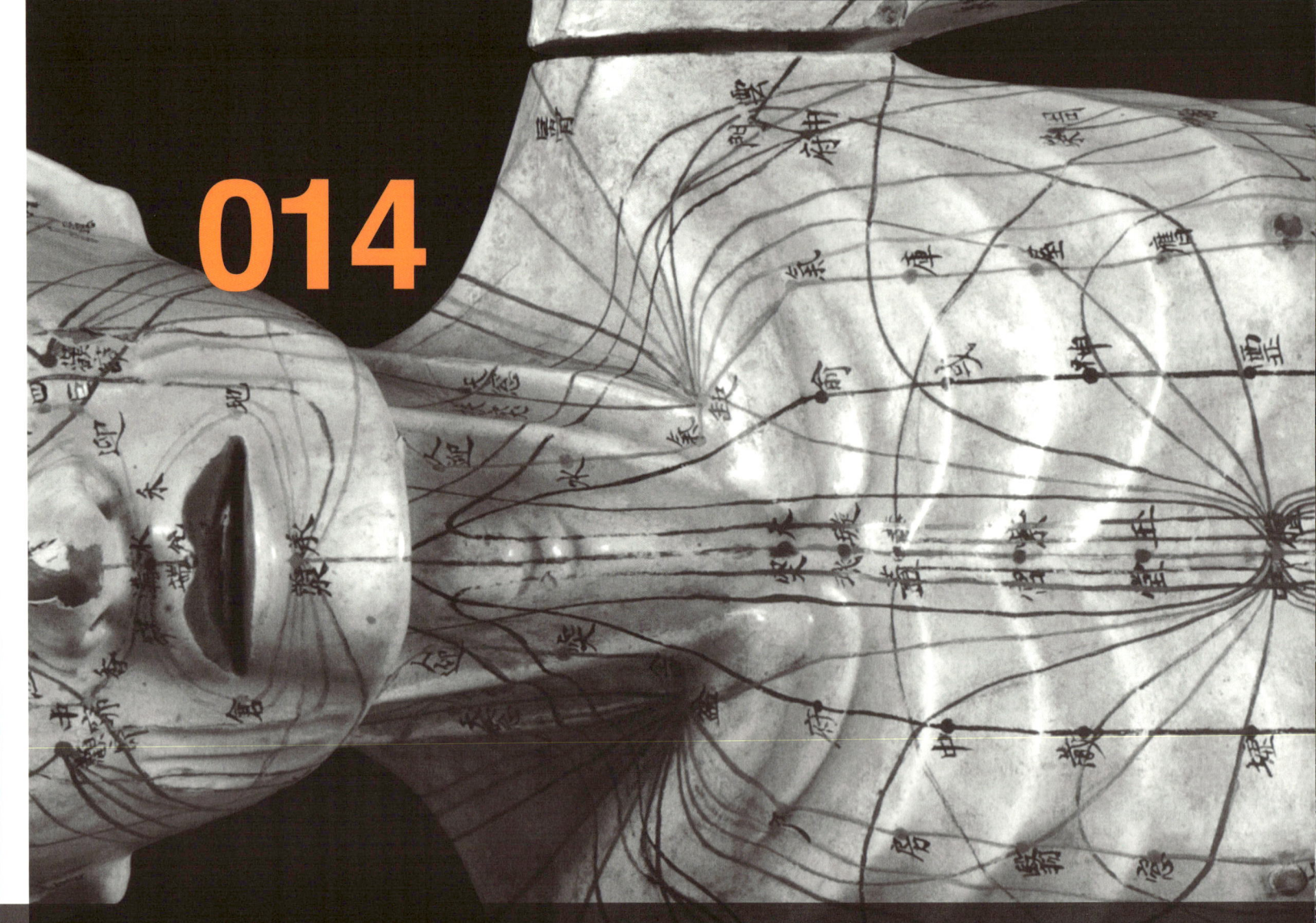

経穴銅人形
慶長年間（1600年前後）／岩田道雪制作／紙塑製、胡粉に上塗り／長870、幅270、高180／東京大学大学院医学系研究科・医学部標本室所蔵

鍼灸治療師の育成に用いられた胴人形である。胴人形という言葉は、中国の「銅人形」に由来する。中国では西暦16年に青銅製の人体模型が作られたとの記録がある。北宋時代の医官で、尚薬奉御となった王惟一（987-1067頃）もまた、仁宋から勅命を受けて天聖5（1027）年に「銅人形」を2体制作し、1体を医官院に、もう1体を大相国寺仁済殿作に奉納している。時代ごと地域ごとの異同があったにせよ、正真のものとされる「銅人形」は、王惟一の著した鍼灸学論『銅人臉穴鍼灸図経』に示される通りの寸法で制作されたようである。胴内は中空で、そこには内臓模型が、頭部と四肢には革袋がそれぞれ収められ、革袋に水銀が充填されていた。体表には経絡経穴説に基づき、365の小孔が穿たれ、14の経路が示されている。「銅人形」は医官の試験に用いられた。受験者は眼を覆い、管針を手に、手探りで所定の経穴を探し当て、小孔に管針を刺入する。もし的を射ていれば袋中の水銀は管針を通って掌中に流れ出て、術者の技の正しいことが示される。もし間違った孔に刺入すると、針が通らぬ仕掛けである。南北朝時代太政大臣の地位にあった藤原公経の子で、僧籍に入った竹田昌慶（1338-1380）が応安2（1369）年に渡明し、中国医学を学び、承和4（1378）年の帰朝のさい、多くの医学書とともに「銅人形」一体を持ち帰った。本品は、中国将来品を基に、慶長年間すなわち1600年前後に、紀州藩の藩医岩田道雪が制作した「経穴胴人形」である。上塗りの上に経穴と経絡が墨で示されている。

Bronze Figure Bearing Acupuncture Points
Around 1600 / Made by Dosetsu Iwata / Paper clay, *gofun* (calcium carbonate) with coating / L870, W270, H180 / Medical Museum, Faculty of Medicine, The University of Tokyo

Used for the education of acupuncturists. The term "bronze figure" originates in China, where we find a record of a human anatomical model made of bronze in A.D. 16. Wang Weiyi (987 – circa 1067), medical officer of the Northern Song dynasty who became court physician, made two bronze figures in 1027 under imperial command, dedicating one to the House of medical officers, and the other to the Daxiangguo Temple. Regardless of the difference in chronology and location, it is said that authentic bronze figures were made according to the dimensions indicated in Wang Weiyi's treaty on acupuncture, *Illustrated Manual for the Practice of Acupuncture and Moxibustion with the Help of a Bronze Figure bearing Acupuncture Points*. Models of internal organs were placed inside the hollow trunk, and leather bags were placed in the cranium and in the limbs. Leather bags were filled with mercury. According to the theory of meridians and acupuncture points, 365 holes were pinned on the surface, and 14 channels indicated. Bronze figures were used during examinations for the grade of medical officer. Candidates were blindfolded and had to feel about the bronze figure to find a given point and insert a needle in it. If they reached the accurate point, the mercury filling the leather bag flew into the palm of their hand through the needle, indicating the exactitude of the practitioner's skill. If the needle was inserted in a wrong point, it did not penetrate the figure. The priest Shokei Takada (1338 – 1380), son of the chancellor of the Nanboku-cho period Fujiwara no Kintsune, travelled to China in 1369 and studied Chinese medicine. Upon his return in 1378, along with numerous medical books, he brought back a bronze figure. The present item is a bronze figure bearing acupuncture points made around 1600 by Dosetsu Iwata, physician of the Kishu Domain, according to the model brought back from China. On the coating, acupuncture points and meridians are indicated in ink.

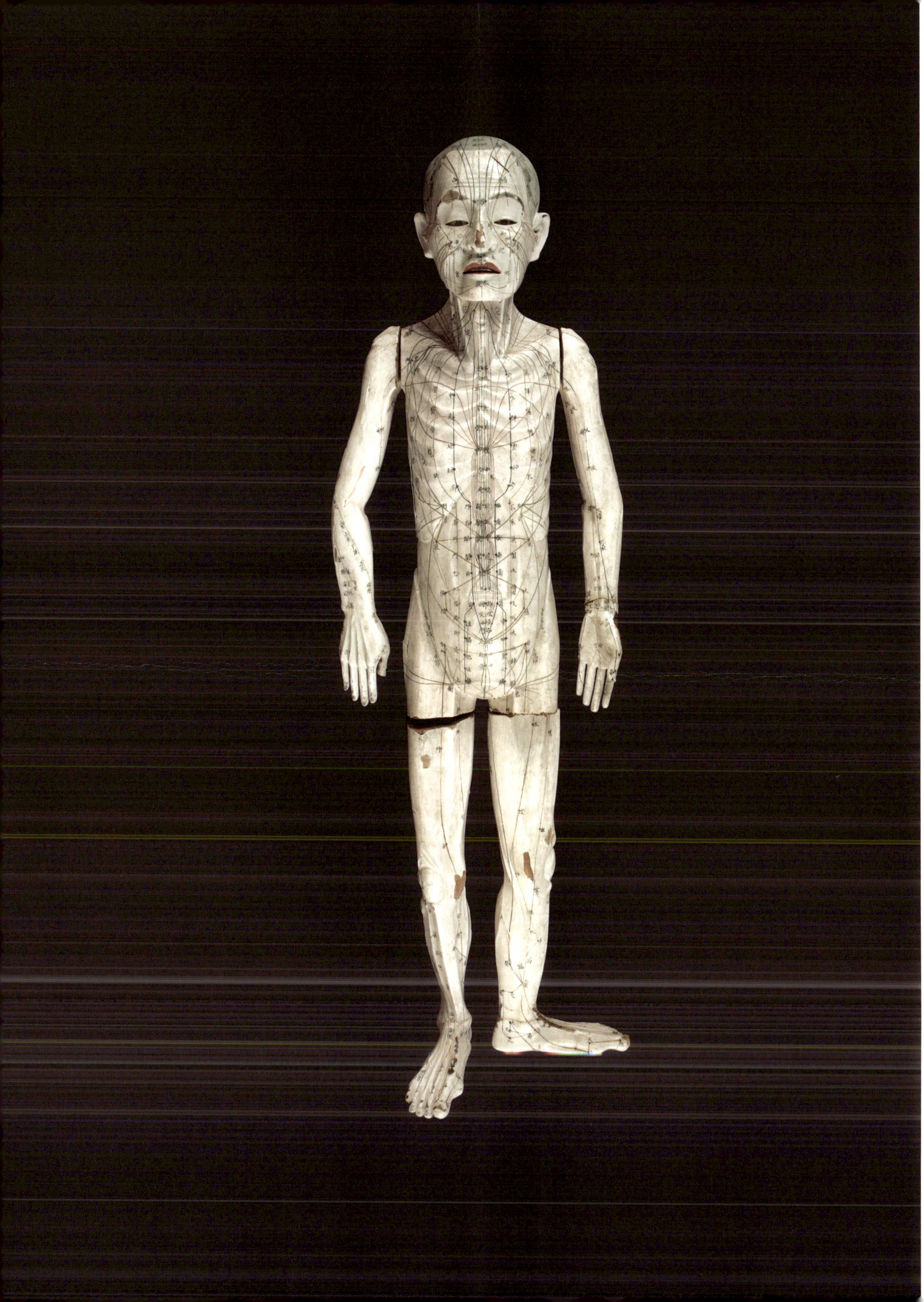

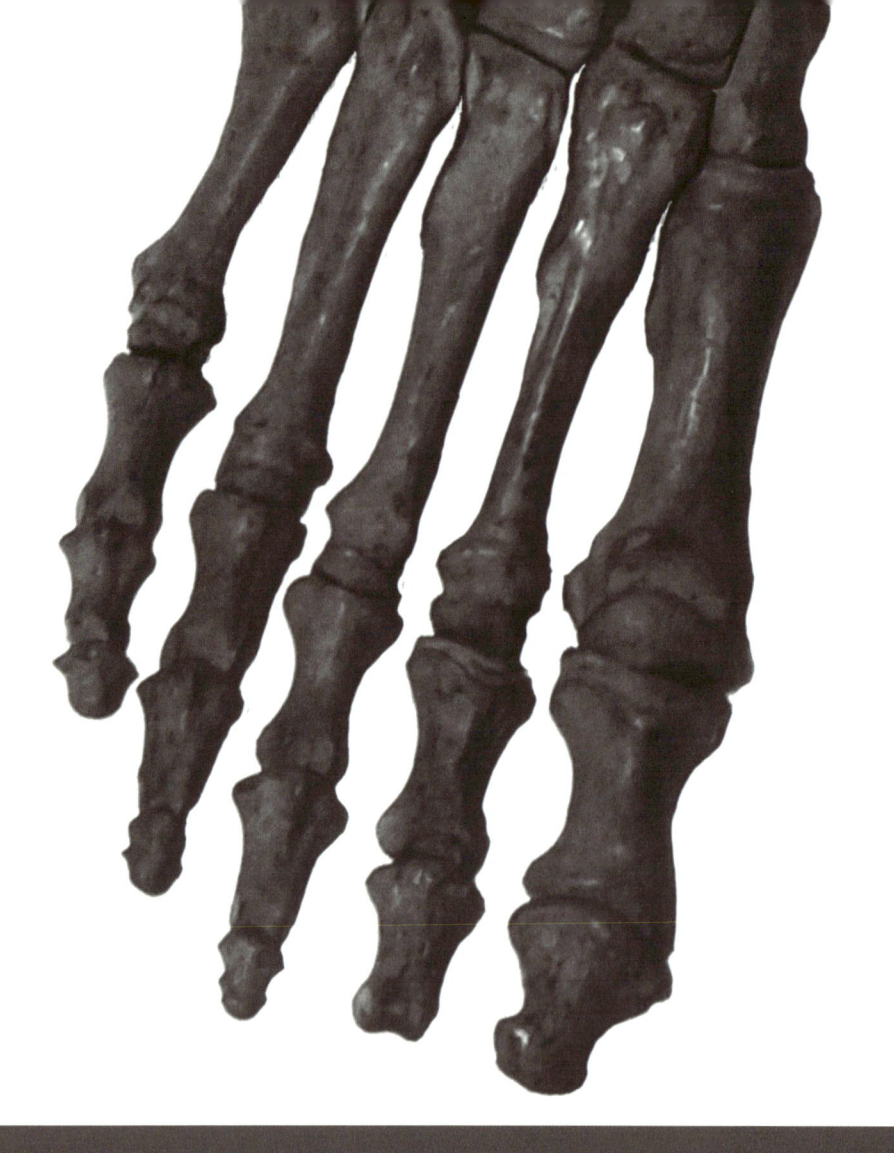

016

木製全身骨格、通称「各務木骨」(頭、脚、手の三部分)

文化7(1810)年頃／各務文献制作／木と紙、胡粉、金属線、竹釘、彩色／全身長2000、幅900、高300／東京大学大学院医学系研究科・医学部標本室所蔵

文化7(1810)年頃、大阪の整骨医各務文献(1765–1829)が、仏師のような彫工に命じて作らせた等身大骨格模型の一部である。制作者の名を取り、「各務木骨」と通称される。文献は本品制作に先立つ2年ほど前にも、もうひとつ別な全身骨格を制作させている。そちらは実物の3分の1に縮体された模型であり、実物大の木骨としては本品が唯一の現存品である。寄せ木を成形し、表面を和紙で整え、その下地に顔料を混ぜた胡粉を塗布し、色を出している。歯の部分には滑石が使われることもあったという。各部の組み立てには、竹釘と針金が使われている。江戸時代には真骨の所持が禁じられていたため、こうした模型が弟子の育成に用いられた。各務文献は実証的な骨学書『整骨新書』の著者であり、文政2(1819)年、木骨とともに自著を幕府医学館へ献納している。文献の献納品は西洋医学所を経て、東校、大学東校から、東京大学医学部へ受け継がれている。明治期にドイツで開かれた博覧会へ出品され、そのさいに四肢の半分と骨盤他の小部分が失われた。

Wooden Full Body Skeleton, Commonly Known as "Kagami Wooden Skeleton" (3 Parts Consisting of the Head, Arm and Hand)

Around 1810 / Made by Bunken Kagami / Wood and paper, *gofun* (calcium carbonate), metallic lines, bamboo nails, coloring / Full body: L2000, W900, H300 / Medical Museum, Faculty of Medicine, The University of Tokyo

This is part of a full-scale skeletal model the osteopath Bunken Kagami (1765 – 1829) had realized around 1810 by a sculptor who could be a Buddhist image maker. It is commonly called "Kagami wooden skeleton," after the maker's name. Two years before the production of the present model, Bunken had another full body skeleton made. That one being a model reduced by one third, the present item is the only extant full-scale wooden skeleton. After modeling structural wooden pieces, the surface was covered with Japanese rice paper, on which coloration consisting of *gofun* powder mixed with pigment was applied. It is said that talc was also used for the teeth. Bamboo nails and wire were used for the assembly. Because the possession of real bones was prohibited during the Edo period, such models were used for the training of students. Bunken Kagami is the author of the demonstrative osteological treatise Osteopathy, which he dedicated in 1819 to the medical institute of the shogunate along with the wooden skeleton. The items dedicated by Bunken were then successively transferred to the Institute of Western Medicine, the Eastern School and the Eastern College before being granted to the Faculty of Medicine of the University of Tokyo. In the Meiji period, the model was shown at an exhibition in Germany, during which half of the limbs as well as small parts of the pelvis were lost.

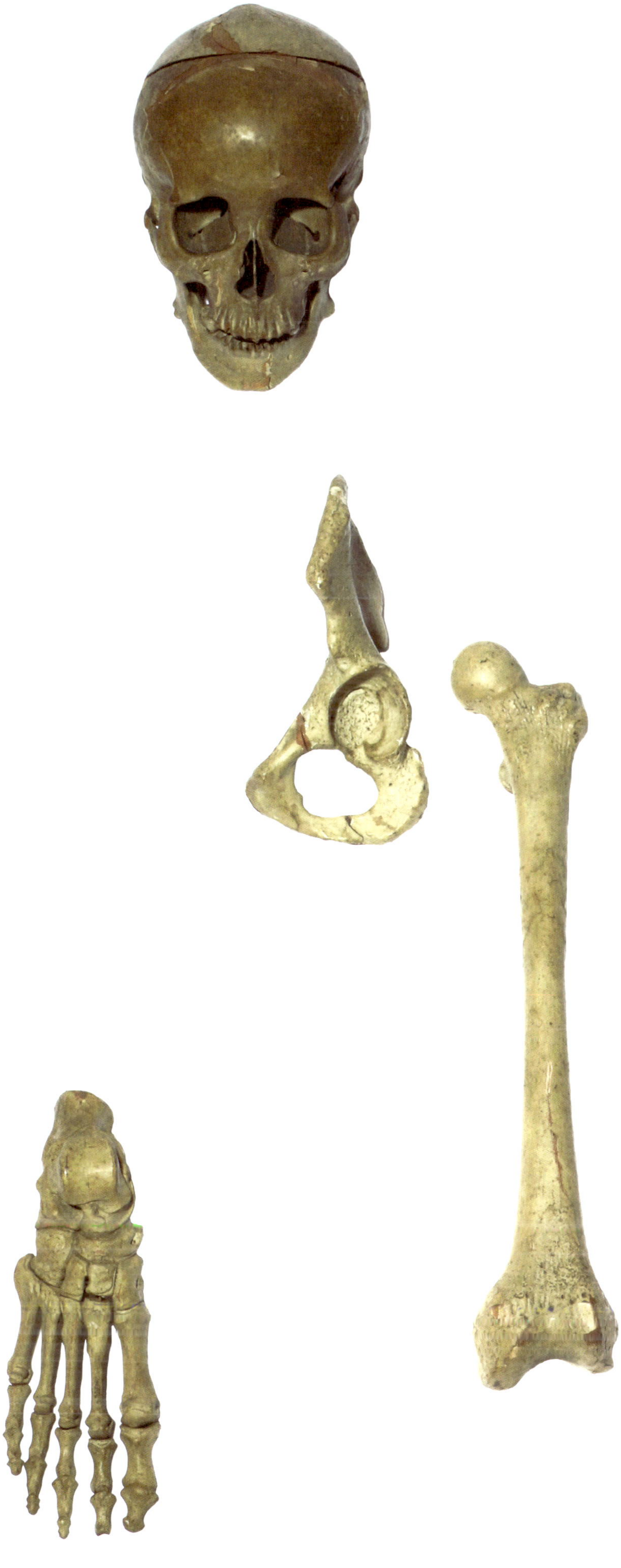

018

徳川御殿医使用治療箱
江戸末期／制作者未詳／金属、木、紙、絹、外箱に蒔絵／外箱縦190、横310、高287、内箱縦180、横302、高280／東京大学大学院医学系研究科・医学部標本室所蔵

江戸末期に御殿医が往診に使っていた薬箱。外箱と内箱の二重構造となっている。内箱の上段には小型の硝子瓶8個と小箱7個が並んで収納されている。15種の薬が揃っており、緊急時に対処できるよう準備されていた。日本では薬を和紙にくるみ、墨で内容を上書きし、小さな抽斗のついた薬箪笥や薬箱に収納しておくというのが伝統的な方法であった。それは東アジアの高温多湿の環境にあって、理に適った薬保存法であった。薬瓶の使用がいつ頃から始まったのかは定かでない。久能山東照宮に徳川家康が薬瓶として使ったとされるガラス瓶が残されているが、これは例外的なもののようで、市井への普及は長崎出島の阿蘭陀商館長がデルフト焼きの薬瓶を持ち込んだことから始まったという。フィリップ・フランツ・フォン・シーボルト（1796–1866）もたくさんの薬瓶を携えて来日している。徳川の御殿医の治療箱には、すでに蘭方医学の処方が取り込まれていたのである。

Medicine Box for the Use of Tokugawa Court Physician
End of the Edo period / Maker unknown / Metal, wood, paper, silk, *maki-e* on outer box / Outer box: L190, W310, H287; Inner box: L180, W302, H280 / Medical Museum, Faculty of Medicine, The University of Tokyo

Medicine box used by court physicians at the end of the Edo period. Has a two-layered structure, including an inner and an outer box. 8 small glass bottles and 7 small boxes are stored in the upper level of the inner box. 15 types of medicine were stored so as to cope with emergencies. In Japan, medicine was traditionally wrapped in Japanese rice paper, on which the contents were written in ink, the package being stored in medicine chests or medicine boxes with small drawers. This conservation method suited the environment of Eastern Asia, marked by high temperature and humidity. It is not certain when medicine bottles started being used. Glass bottles said to have been used as medicine bottles by Ieyasu Tokugawa remain at the Kunozan Toshogu, but they seem to be rather exceptional. Their generalized use started with the introduction of Delftware medicine bottles by the director of the Dutch trading post at Dejima, Nagasaki. Philipp Franz von Siebold (1796-1866) came to Japan carrying many medicine bottles. Dutch medical methods were thus already implemented in medicine boxes used by the Tokugawa court physicians.

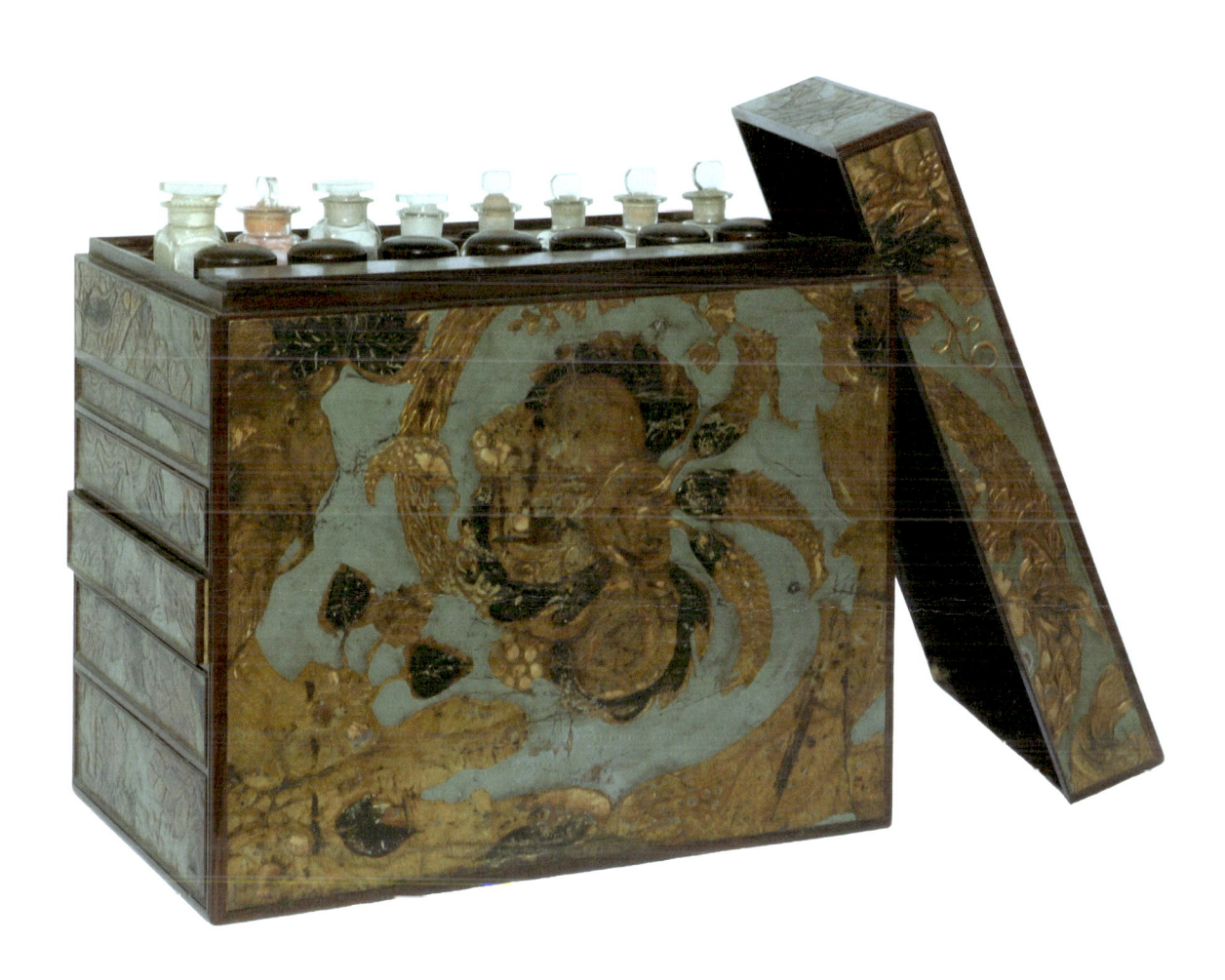

020

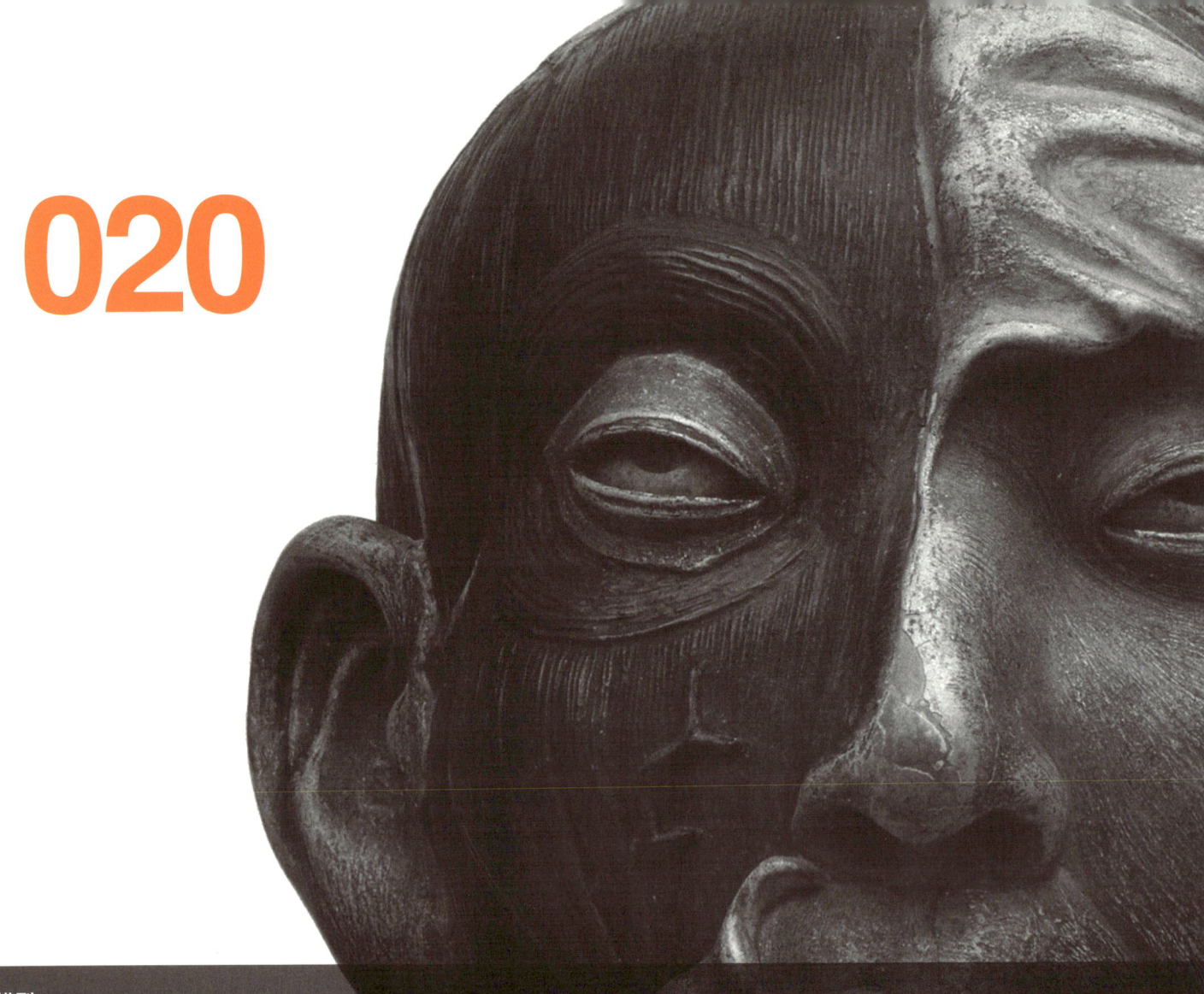

人頭解剖模型
寛政6(1794)年／鈴木常八制作（桂川甫周の注文による）／桧の寄せ木材に胡粉、彩色／長215、幅155、高215／東京大学医学部解剖学教室旧蔵（桂川家旧蔵）／大学院医学系研究科・医学部標本室所蔵

後頭部内面に「作之　鈴木常八　寛政　寅十月」の墨書がある。寛政6(1794)年5月和蘭陀商館長ヘンミイが医師ケラーの随伴で江戸参府を果たしたさい、日本の蘭学者に贈ったフランス製蝋細工模型を基に、幕府官医桂川甫周(1754–1809)が職人鈴木常八を使って制作させたもの。国産桧を寄せ木し、胡粉の地塗りの上に岩絵具で彩色が施してある。肌色の部分には、近世の能面に見られる刷毛眼塗り技法が使われている。歯は獣骨ないし角から彫り出されている。両眼には、仏像と同様、ガラスによる玉眼がはめ込まれている。頭の表皮を剥ぎ、浅層筋と静脈を表現している。明治初年、桂川家が織田信徳へ譲渡し、明治22(1889)年1月に織田が東京大学医学部に寄贈したことが、附属資料から確認できる。昭和52(1977)年、西川杏太郎・中里寿克による全面的な修復がなされている。

Anatomical Model of Human Head
1794 / Made by Tsunehachi Suzuki (upon Hoshu Katsuragawa's order) / Assembled pieces of Japanese cypress, *gofun* (calcium carbonate) and coloring / L215, W155, H215 / Former collection of the Laboratory of Anatomy, Faculty of Medicine, The University of Tokyo (former collection of the Katsuragawa family) / Medical Museum, Faculty of Medicine, The University of Tokyo

The back of the head, in its inner part, bears the inscription in Japanese in ink "Made by Tsunehachi Suzuki in Winter of the Kansei period." The shogunate physician Hoshu Katsuragawa (1754 – 1809) had it made by the craftsman Tsunehachi Suzuki, based on the French-made wax model given to Japanese scholars in Dutch studies by G. Hemmij, director of the Dutch trading post, upon his visit to the Edo government in May 1794 in company of physician A.L.B. Keller. On assembled pieces of Japanese cypress, *gofun* powder is applied, colored with natural mineral pigments. For the flesh-colored parts, the brush-marking lacquering technique known as *hakeme-nuri*, used on modern *no* masks, is applied. Teeth are carved out of animal bones and horns. For both eyes, glass balls are fitted in, as for Buddhist sculptures. Outer muscles and veins are expressed by stripping off the head epidermis. Attached documentation testifies that this was passed on in the beginning of the Meiji period by the Katsuragawa family to Nobunori Oda, who in turn donated it to the Faculty of Medicine of the University of Tokyo in January 1889. In 1977, it was fully restored by Kyotaro Nishikawa and Toshikatsu Nakazato.

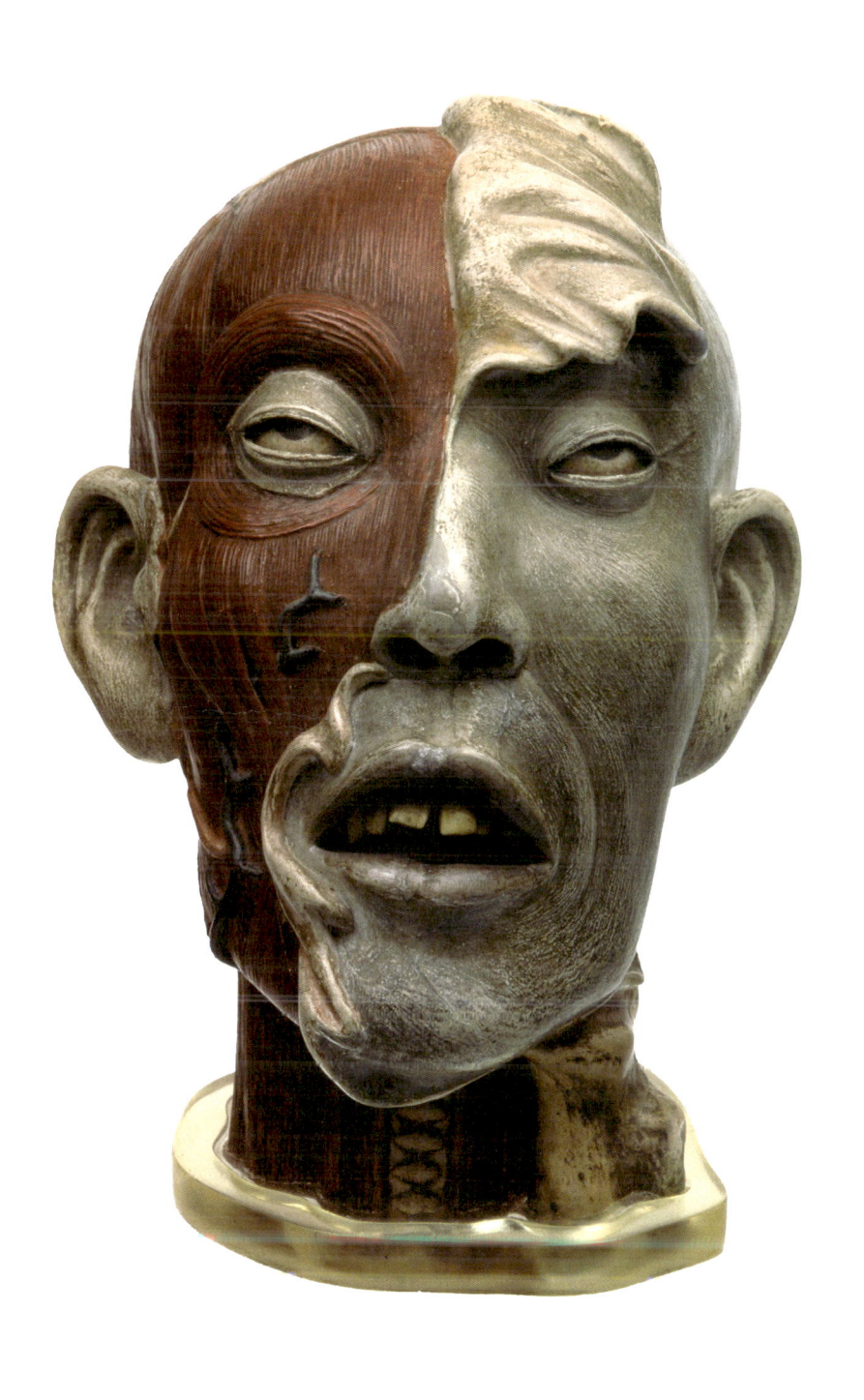

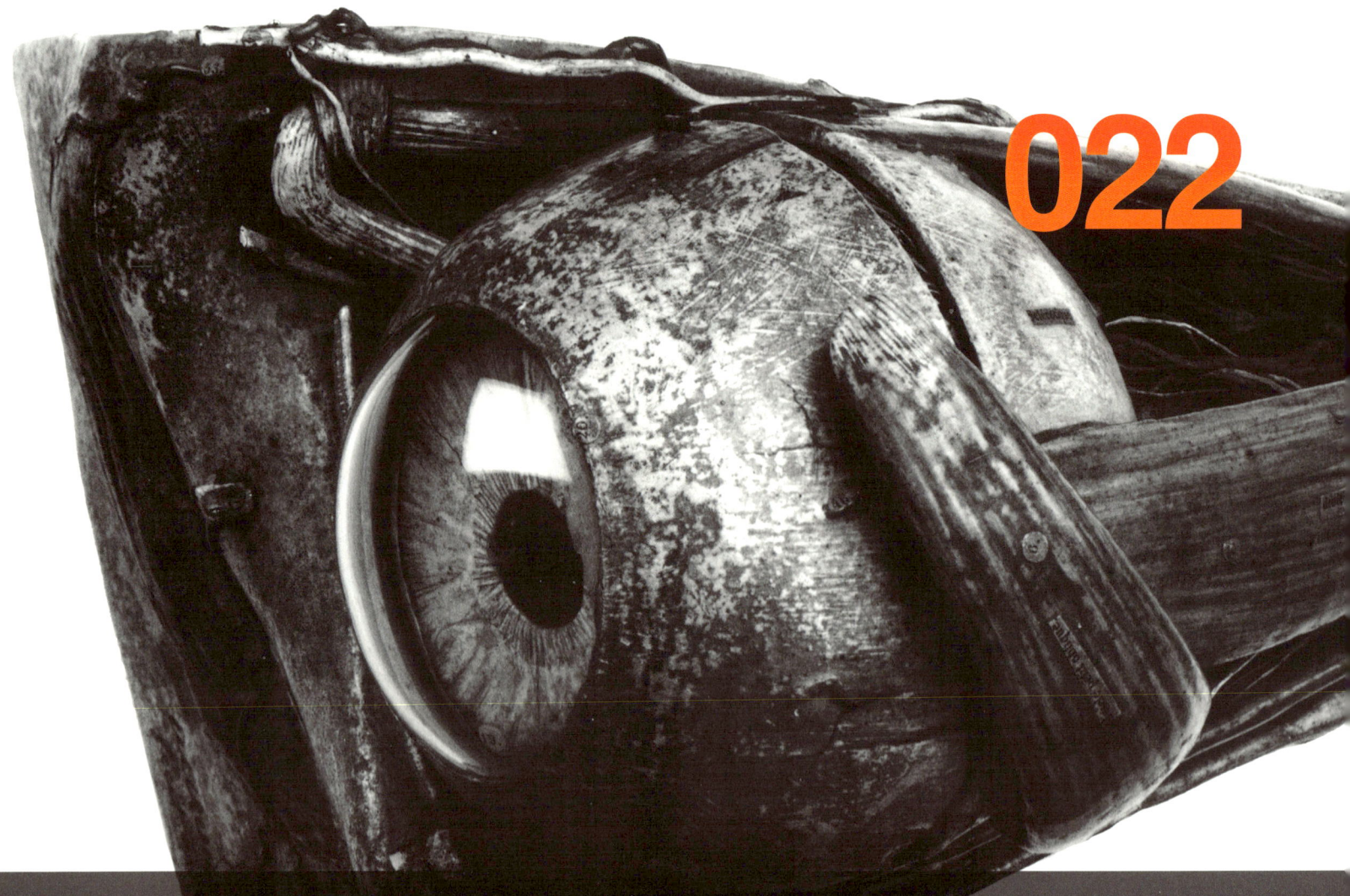

眼球解剖模型

文久3(1863)年／ルイ・トマ・ジェローム・オズー制作／紙粘土、ガラス／縦285、横175、高200／東京大学医学部眼科学教室旧蔵(伊東玄伯購入・旧蔵)／大学院医学系研究科・医学部標本室所蔵

長崎の医学伝習所でオランダ人軍医ポンペ・ファン・メールデルフォールト(1829–1908)について眼科学を学び、安政4(1857)年11月、師の帰国にさいし幕府の最初の留学生として、オランダへ渡った伊東玄伯(1832–1898)がヨーロッパで購入したものである。「オズー博士、一八六三年」の記載があることから、文久3(1863)年に医師ルイ・トマ・ジェローム・オズー(1797–1880)の制作したものであることがわかる。乾燥標本、液浸標本、蝋製ムラージュ、皮剥エコルシェなど、医学教育研究用の各種標本教材のなかにあって、紙粘土製人体模型標本は「キンストレーキ」と呼ばれ、開発されて間のない、当時としては最新の研究教材であった。玄伯は1867年のパリ万国博覧会のためフランスに滞留していた幕府名代徳川昭武(1853–1910)を表敬訪問すべく、同年5月にパリを訪れており、そのさい最新式模型標本を入手したものと思われる。玄伯は明治元(1868)年の帰朝のさいに、これを日本に持ち帰っている。なお、「キンストレーキ」については、ポンペが万延元(1860)年にパリから取り寄せたもの、竹内下野守保徳(1807–1867)率いる文久2(1862)年遣欧使節団が持ち帰ったものが知られており、それらはいずれもオズーの制作品だったと考えられる。本標本は、左眼球と眼筋の構造を示すもので、大きさは実物の約10倍に相当する。玄伯自筆の年記が前部にオランダ語で記されている。玄伯は後に方成を名乗り、侍医となった。没後、『通俗百歳長寿法——食養衛生』(東京 二松堂、1911年刊)の著者として知られる菊地武恒の手に渡り、後に令息の菊地武信(当時陸軍軍医学校教官)から、本学医学部眼科学教室へ寄贈された。

Anatomical Model of Eyeball

1863 / Made by Louis Thomas Jérôme Auzoux / Paper clay, glass / L285, W175, H200 / Former collection of the Laboratory of Ophthalmology, Faculty of Medicine, The University of Tokyo (Acquired and formerly owned by Genpaku Ito) / Medical Museum, Faculty of Medicine, The University of Tokyo

This was bought in Europe by Genpaku Ito (1832 – 1898) when he travelled to the Netherlands as the shogunate's first overseas student in November 1857. This coincided with the return of his instructor, the Dutch medical officer Johannes Lijdius Catharinus Pompe van Meerdervoort (1829 – 1908), under whom he had studied ophthalmology at the Nagasaki Medical Training Institute. The inscription "Auzoux Doct.er fecit anno 1863" certifies that this was made by doctor Louis Thomas Jérôme Auzoux (1797 - 1880) in 1863. When compared to each type of educational model employed in medical research and education such as dry specimens, wet specimens, wax models and *écorchés*, the technique of human body models made of paper clay and called *clastique* had just been developed: it was then the most advanced type of research material. As he had to pay a courtesy visit to Akitake Tokugawa (1853 – 1910) who was staying in Paris on behalf of the shogunate for the International Exposition of 1867, Genpaku Ito went to Paris in May of the same year, and it is thought that he acquired the newest models and specimens then. Upon his return in 1868, Genpaku brought this back to Japan. As far as *clastique* models are concerned, those ordered by Pompe from Paris in 1860, and those brought back by the 1862 delegation led by Yasunori Takeuchi (1807 – 1867) are known, all of which are thought to have been made by Auzoux. The present specimen represents the structure of the left eyeball and ocular muscles, and is ten times bigger than the original. The year is written by hand in Dutch by Genpaku himself. Genpaku, who later went by the name of Hosei, became a court physician. After his death, the model was in the hands of Taketsune Kikuchi, known as the author of *Popular methods of longevity: food hygiene* (published in Tokyo by Nishodo in 1911). His son Takenobu Kikuchi, then teaching at the Military Medical College, eventually donated it to the Laboratory of Ophthalmology of the Faculty of Medicine.

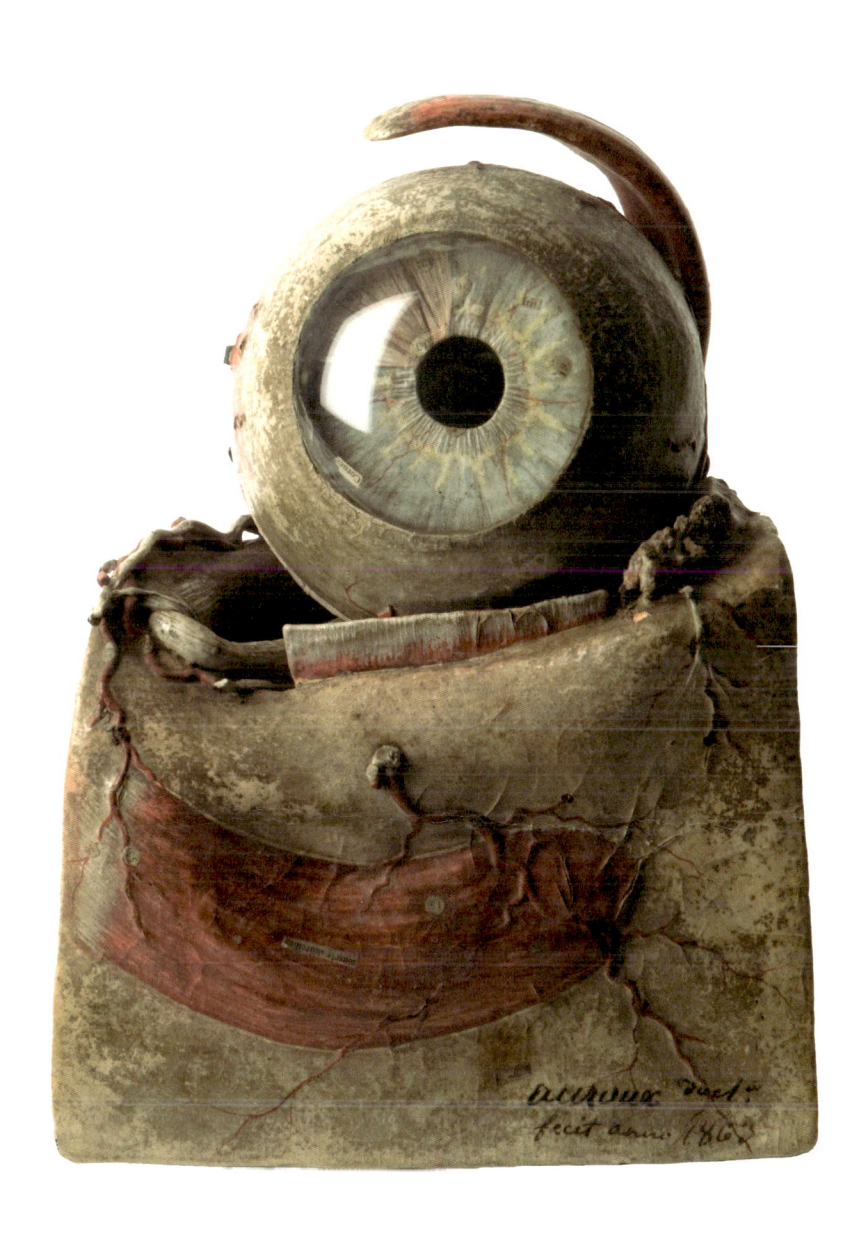

024

オランダ人頭蓋骨（医学部第一号標本）
19世紀前半／骨縦200、横140、台縦235、横180、高30／ポンペ・ファン・メールデルフォールト旧蔵、軍医総監松本良順寄贈／東京大学大学院医学系研究科・医学部標本室所蔵

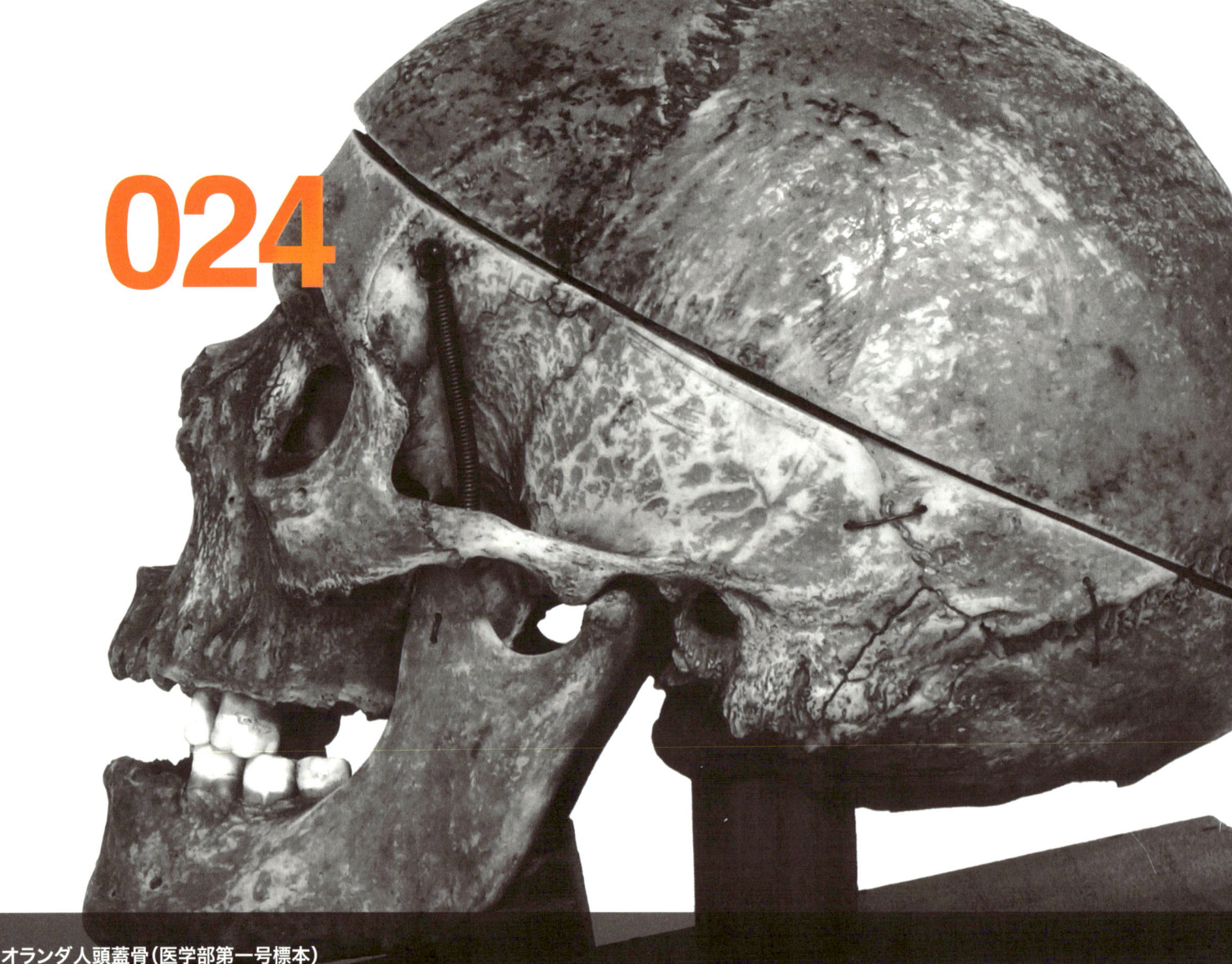

明治時代に整理された東京大学医学部解剖学教室の『解剖学標本台帳』によると、第一号標本は「オランダ人頭蓋骨」とされ、その備考欄に「軍医総監松本良順氏の寄贈」と記録されている。松本良順（1832-1907）は長崎の医学伝習所において、西洋式医学を導入しようとするオランダ人軍医ポンペ・ファン・メールデルフォールト（1829-1907）について学び、その助手となった。当時の日本人として、もっとも本格的に西洋近代医学を修めたのが松本良順だったのである。松本は長崎の医学伝習所から江戸の西洋医学所へ召還され、緒方洪庵（1810-1863）の後任として、三代目頭取を務めることになった。会津戦争で幕府軍の傷病兵の治療に奔走したことから、幕府瓦解後、投獄され、1年間を獄中で過ごすことになった。明治6（1873）年には、陸軍卿山形有朋（1838-1922）の要請で初代軍医総監に就任した。ポンペは解剖学を講じるにあたって、献体によるとされたオランダ人頭蓋骨を教材として使ったと言われ、良順が長崎を離れるとき、その頭蓋骨を愛弟子に記念として贈った。江戸に戻った良順は、西洋医学所でポンペ譲りの頭蓋骨を用いて教育にあたった。当時、その頭蓋骨が医学生たちにとっていかに貴重な教材であったか、「実物を知りたい学生達でひっぱり凧となり、手垢で黒光りして、まるで漆を塗ったようになった」と、のちに軍医総監となる石黒忠悳（1845-1941）が昭和11（1936）年に博文館から刊行した私家本『懐旧九十年』のなかで証言している。

Skull of a Dutchman (First Specimen of the Faculty of Medicine)
First half of the 19th Century / Skull: L200, W140; Base: L235, W180, H30 / Former collection of Pompe van Meerdervoort, donated by Ryojun Matsumoto / Medical Museum, Faculty of Medicine, The University of Tokyo

According to the *Register of Anatomical Specimens* edited by the Laboratory of Anatomy of the Faculty of Medicine of the University of Tokyo during the Meiji period, the first specimen is the "skull of a Dutchman" and the additional remarks column states: "donated by Ryojun Matsumoto, Surgeon General of the Army." Ryojun Matsumoto (1832 – 1907) learned at the Nagasaki Medical Training Institute under Dutch medical officer Pompe van Meerdervoort (1829 – 1907), who was then trying to introduce Western medicine, eventually becoming his assistant. As a Japanese then, it is Ryojun Matsumoto who had the most complete training in Western modern medicine. Matsumoto was recalled from the Nagasaki Medical Training Institute to the Western Medical Institute in Edo, where he served as the third director, succeeding to Koan Ogata (1810 – 1863). Having worked to cure the sick and wounded of the shogunate army during the Battle of Aizu, he was imprisoned after the collapse of the shogunate, and spent one year in prison. In 1873, upon the request of Aritomo Yamagata (1838 – 1922), he was named first Surgeon General of the Army. When teaching, Pompe is said to have used the skull of a Dutchman issued from a body donation as an education material, and he gave it to Ryojun as a souvenir when his disciple left Nagasaki. Having returned to Edo, Ryojun used Pompe's skull for educational purposes at the Western Medical Institute. Testifying to the preciousness of that skull in the eyes of the medical students of the time, Tadanori Ishiguro (1845 – 1941), who later became Surgeon General of the Army, writes in *Reminiscing Ninety Years*, his privately published book (Hakubunkan, 1936): "It was in great demand among students wanting to know the real object, getting thumbed to the point of being covered with black luster, as if it had been lacquered."

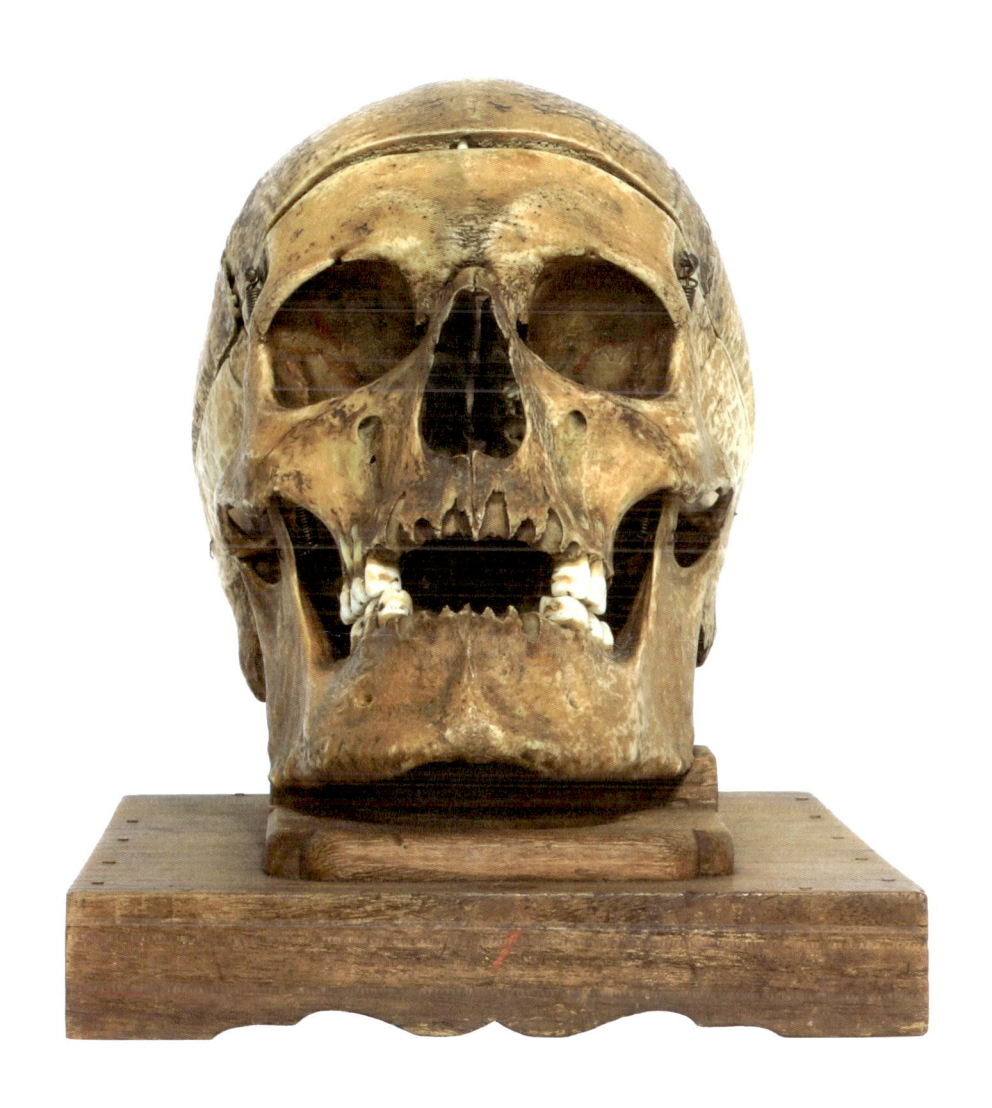

026

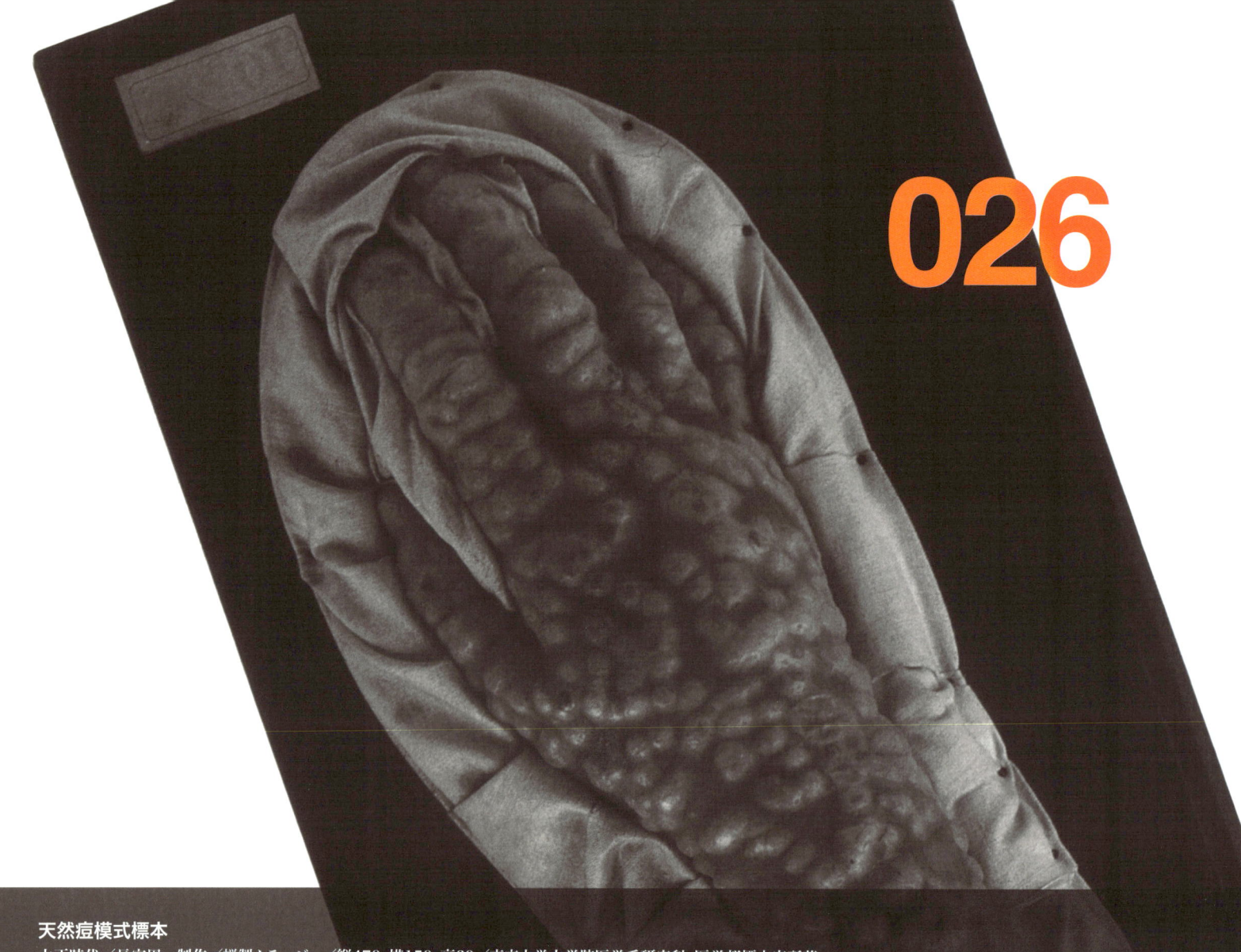

天然痘模式標本
大正時代／長安周一制作／蝋製ムラージュ／縦470、横150、高60／東京大学大学院医学系研究科・医学部標本室所蔵

蝋を人体を型どって作る蝋製ムラージュは、皮膚科疾患の記録用に長く役立てられてきた。現代ではデジタル画像による症例記録が実用化されているが、ひとむかし前までムラージュ標本が医学教育研究の現場で有用視されていたのである。皮膚疾患の患部に油を塗り、石膏を流して雌型を取る。これにパラフィンと蝋の混合物を流し込み、得られた雄型に彩色を施したものがムラージュである。これを国内に導入したのは、明治31（1898）年から大正15（1926）年まで、医学部皮膚科学・泌尿器科学の教授を務めた土肥慶蔵（1866-1931）である。土肥はヨーロッパ留学時代にムラージュ標本の有用性を認識し、ウィーン大学のカポシー教授の許でその技術を学び、帰国後、国内での普及に努め、伊藤有、長安周一ら、ムラージュ制作の名匠を育てた。「天然痘ムラージュ模式標本」は、昭和55（1980）年の根絶宣言をもって病気それ自体が地球上から完全に駆逐されたとされているため、本品のような代替標本を通してしか症状を観察することができない。現在ではほとんど見られなくなった珍しい疾患を記録したムラージュ標本が、医学系研究科・医学部標本室と総合研究博物館資料部医学部門の2ヶ所に、あわせて500点ほど残されている。

Model Specimen of Smallpox
Taisho period / Made by Shuichi Nagayasu / Wax moulage / L470, W150, H60 / Medical Museum, Graduate School of Medicine and Faculty of Medicine, The University of Tokyo

Wax moulages, made by applying wax to the human body, were long useful as a recording device of skin diseases. The recording of medical cases according to digital imagery is now put in practice, but until quite recently, moulage specimens were regarded as being efficient for medical education and research. The mold was made by applying oil on the body part affected by a skin disease, and by pouring plaster. A composite of paraffin and wax was then cast in, and coloring was applied to the obtained form to create the moulage. This technique was introduced in Japan by Keizo Dohi (1866 – 1931), who served as professor of Dermatology and Urology at the Faculty of Medicine from 1898 to 1926. Dohi perceived the importance of moulage specimens during his study years in Europe, learning the technique under Professor Kaposi of the University of Vienna. After his return to Japan, he worked for its generalization, training master fabricants of moulage such as Yu Ito and Shuichi Nagayasu. With the announcement of the eradication of smallpox in 1980, the disease itself having been extirpated from the surface of the Earth, it is now only possible to observe its symptoms through substitutes such as the present moulage specimen. The Medical Museum of the Graduate School of Medicine and Faculty of Medicine and the Medicine Section of the Research Materials Department of the University Museum hold together about 50 of such moulage specimens, which record rare diseases having now almost disappeared.

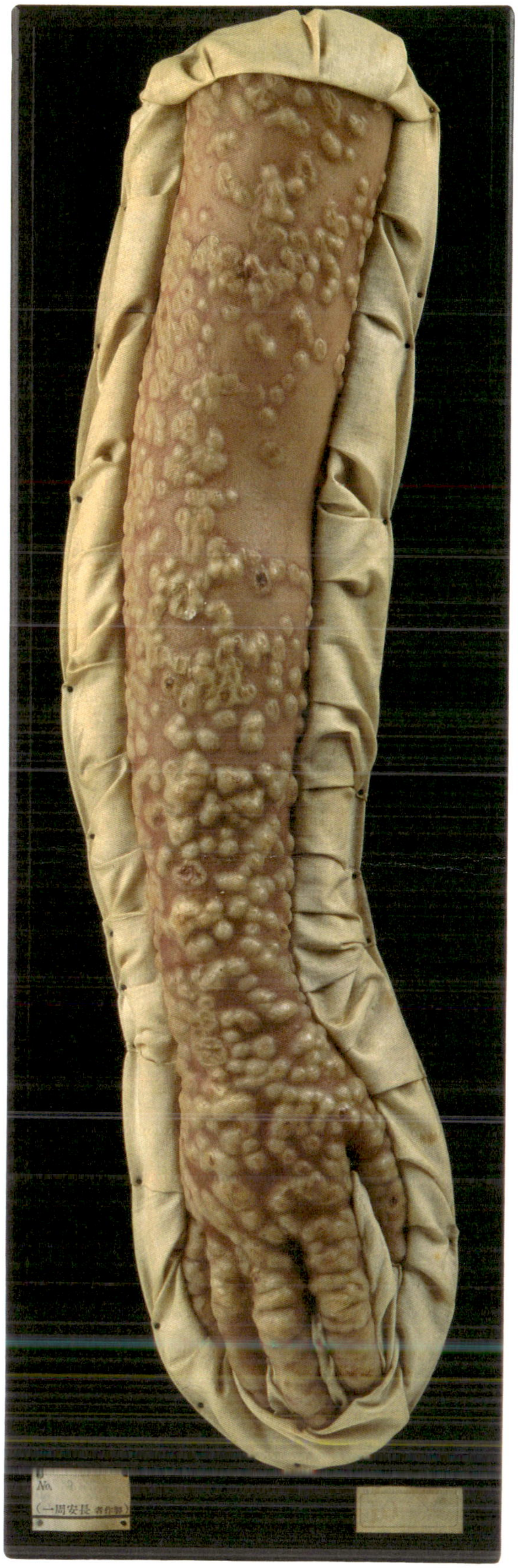

028

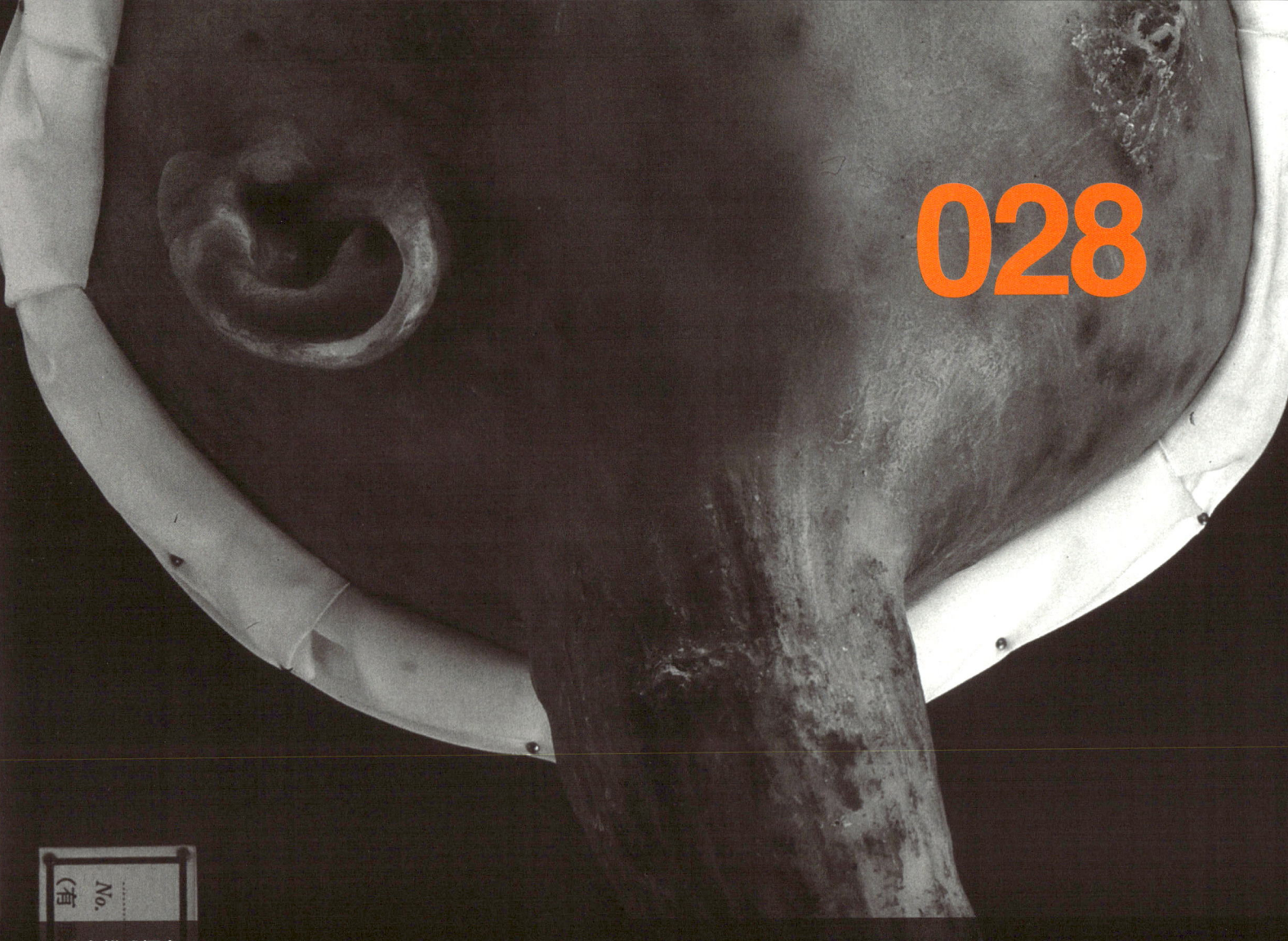

皮角模式標本
大正時代／伊藤有制作／蠟製ムラージュ／縦255、横385、高130／東京大学大学院医学系研究科・医学部標本室所蔵

土肥慶蔵（1866-1931）が育てたムラージュ職人伊藤有の手になる。中国で見いだされた特異な症例である。言葉による説明では容易に納得し難い現実も、こうした症例標本をもってすれば一目瞭然である。なお、ムラージュ標本に使われる蠟は、モノの表面を転写するのに向いているが、破損すると補修し難いという難点もある。

Model Specimen of Cutaneous Horn
Taisho period / Made by Yu Ito / Wax moulage / L255, W385, H130 / Medical Museum, Graduate School of Medicine and Faculty of Medicine, The University of Tokyo

Specimen made by Yu Ito, the moulage artisan trained by Keizo Dohi (1866 – 1931). This is a unique pathological case discovered in China. A reality which can hardly be understood through verbal explanations suddenly becomes strikingly evident with the use of such case specimens. The wax used in moulage specimens is suited to transfer the surface of things, but its drawback is that it can hardly be repaired when broken.

皮 角

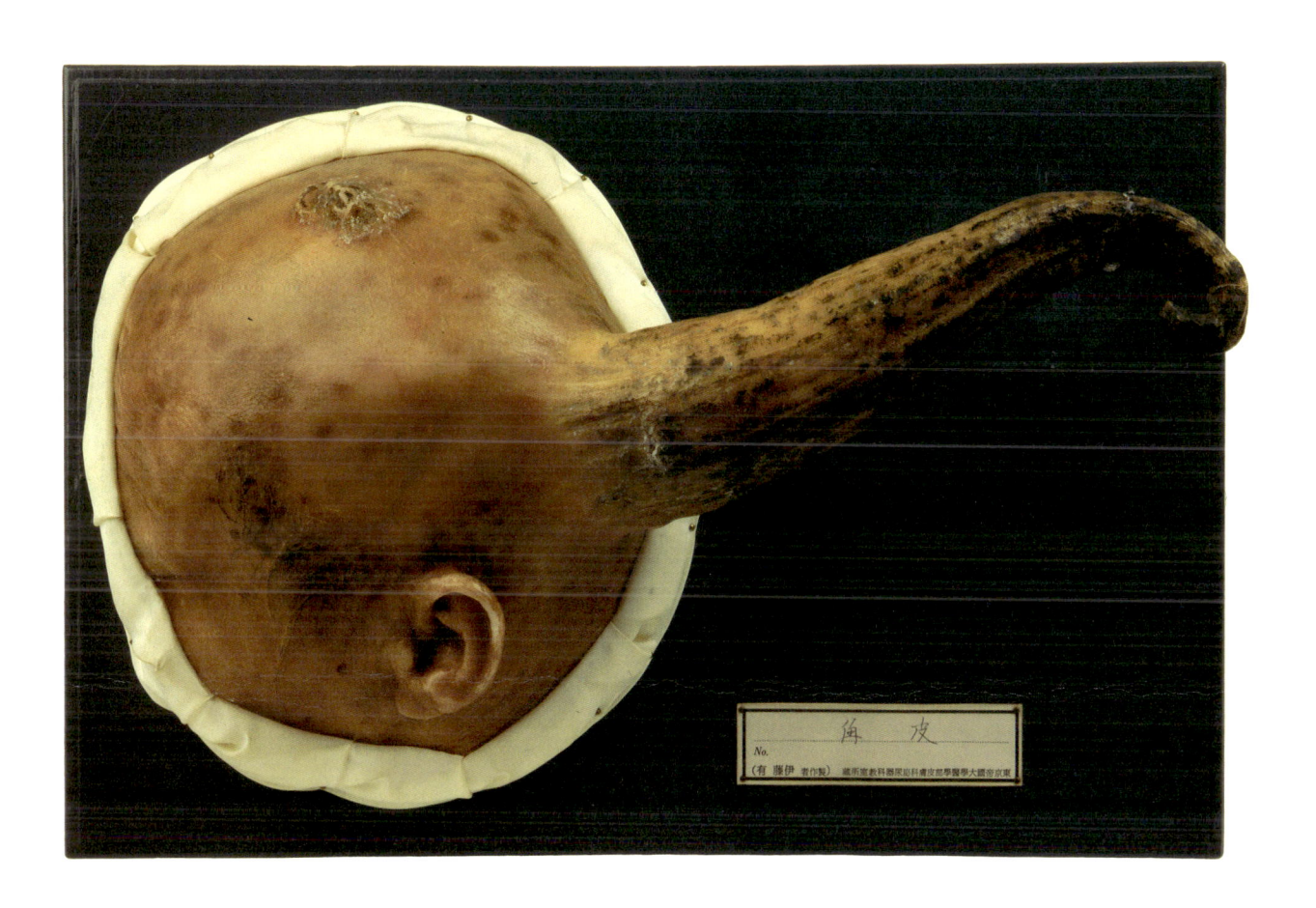

東京帝國大學醫學部皮膚科黴毒科教室藏　（伊藤 著作者　有）

030

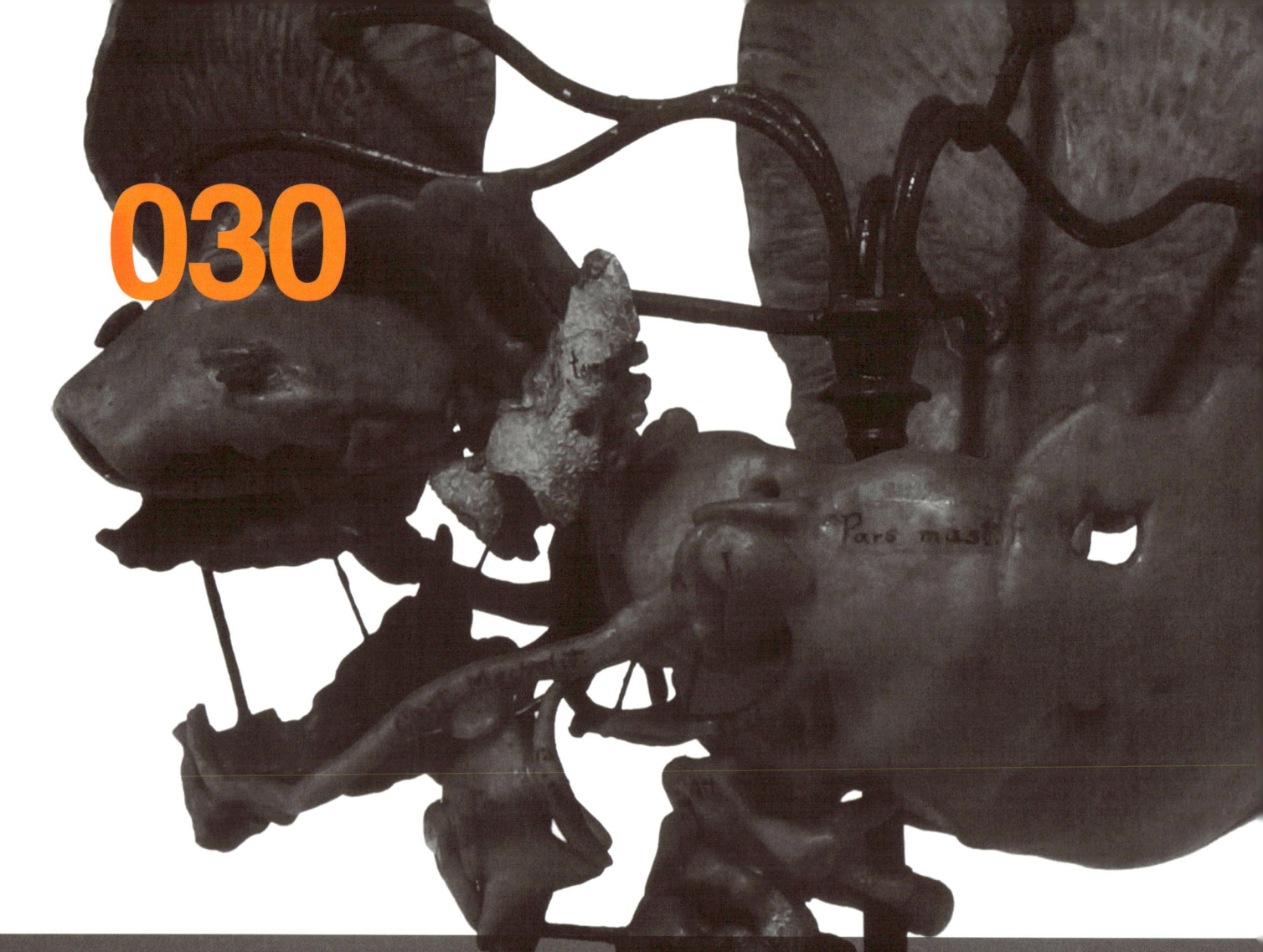

頭蓋発生模型
年代未詳／蝋製に木製台座／縦325、横220、奥230／東京大学大学院医学系研究科・医学部標本室所蔵

事物や事象を観察し、構造やシステムを理解する。これがサイエンスの基本である。成長を続ける生命体の場合には、発生や成長のプロセスを時系列にそって段階的に示すセット標本が、理解を助ける上で重宝である。そのため、発生模型は医学標本の定番となった。

Model of Cranial Development
Date unknown / Wax, wooden base / L325, W220, H230 / Medical Museum, Graduate School of Medicine and Faculty of Medicine, The University of Tokyo

Observing things and phenomena, and understanding their structure and system: such is the basis of science. In the case of living organisms which continually grow, sets of specimens which chronologically represent each step of a development or growth process are particularly precious in that they help comprehension. This is why development models became standard among medical specimens.

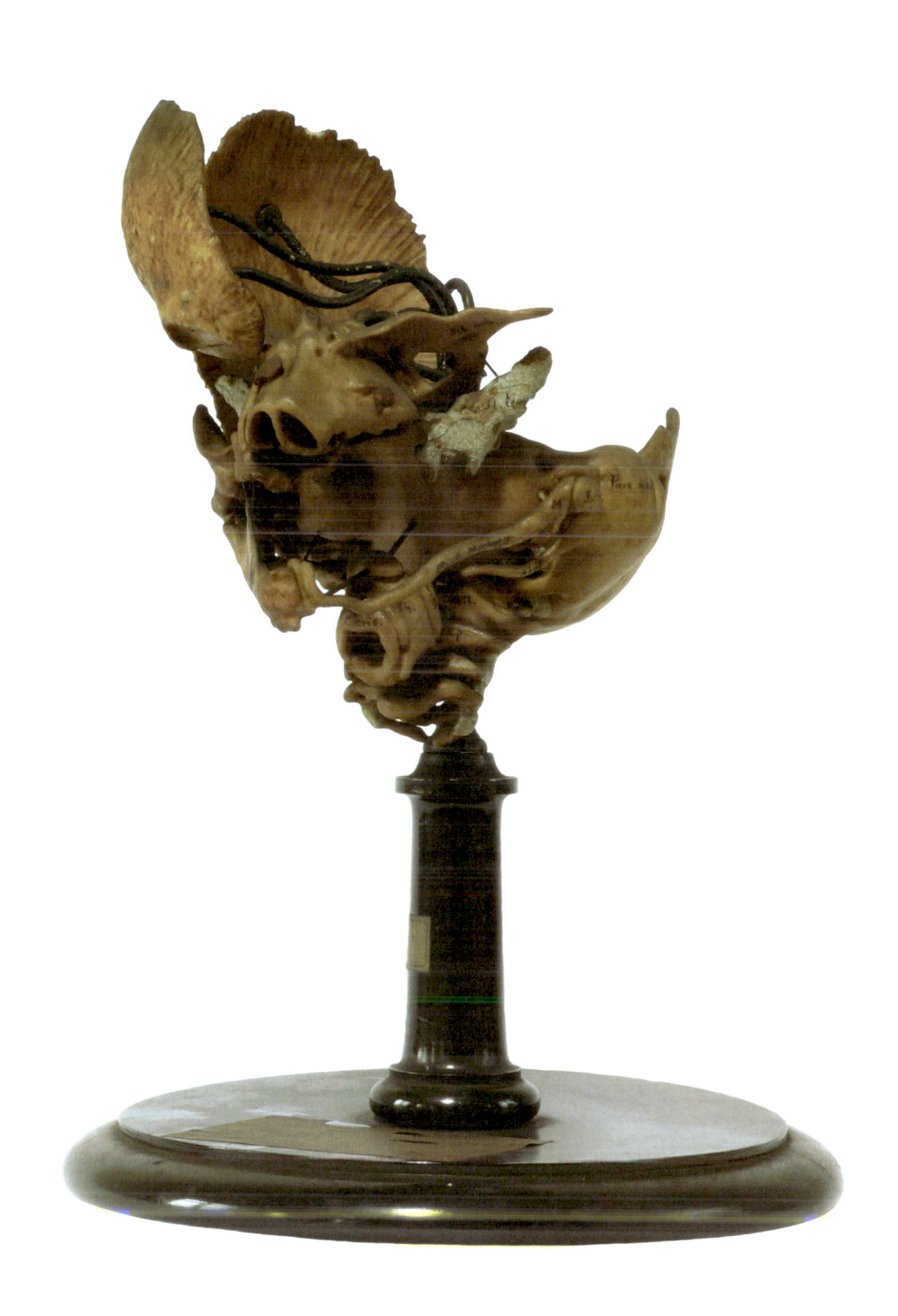

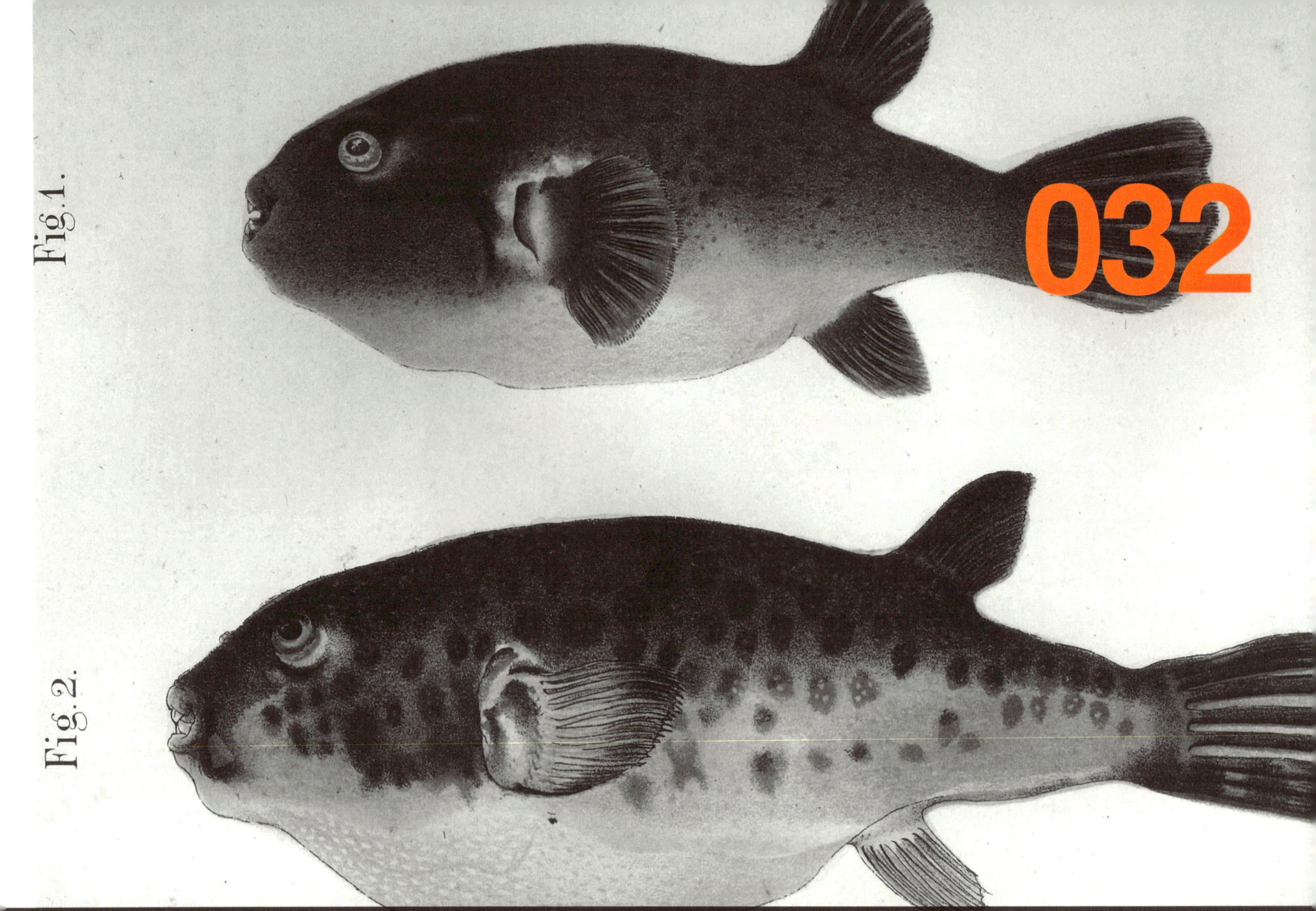

Fig.1.

Fig.2.

032

『帝国大学紀要医科』第1冊第5号
明治25(1892)年／帝国大学印行／冊子本／縦260、横142／東京大学医学部薬理学教室旧蔵／総合研究博物館研究部所蔵

明治12(1879)年に理学部から出版された『理科会粋(メモア)』は国内初の研究紀要として知られるが、当初は御雇外国人の研究成果を国外へ報告するためのものであった。日本人の業績がそこに収載されるようになったのは、明治15(1882)年以降のことである。他の部局が同様の紀要を創刊するのはさらに遅く、東京帝国大学へ改組されてから後のことになる。その先駆けのひとつが『帝国大学紀要医科』であった。同紀要の創刊号には医科大学教授の著名な論文が並んでいる。最高級の舶来用紙にすべて欧文で印刷されており、図版は石版による。画工の手で手彩色の施された折り込み図版も多い。本図は薬物学教授の職にあった高橋順太郎(1856-1920)のフグ毒研究に附された図版である。ベルリンとストラスブールで薬物学を学んだ高橋は、明治18(1885)年10月末に帰国し、翌月から東京大学御用掛に任ぜられ、医科大学専任講師として薬物学を講じることになった。国内ではテオドール・ホフマン(1837-1894)、エルヴィン・フォン・ベルツ(1849-1913)、印東玄得(1850-1895)らが、内科講義の傍らに薬物論を講じてきた。そうした学史的過去を振り返るなら、高橋が教授に就任した明治19(1886)年を、薬物学教室の創設年と見なすことができる。高橋の業績でよく知られるのが、助教授猪子吉人(1866-1893)と共同でなされた、フグ毒の生理的作用に関する研究である。研究に着手したのは、留学から戻って2年後の明治20(1887)年のことであった。これが動物試験を基にした実験薬理学の端緒を拓くことになる。フグ毒は生魚の体内にあり、水にも解け易い。そのことから、高橋はフグ毒素がタンパク質系のものでないことを証明し、「毒力表」なるものを作成してみせた。本図は魚体の部分にアラビアゴムの層が敷かれている。そのため、体表のヌメリ感が見事に再現されることとなった。かくも見事な印刷が実現し得たのは、帝大医科の権威の高さの故であった。

The Imperial University Bulletin of Medical Science, Vol. 1, No. 5
1892 / Published by the Imperial University / Booklet / L260, W142 / Former collection of the Laboratory of Pharmacology, Faculty of Medicine, The University of Tokyo / Research Department, UMUT

The *Memoirs of the Science Department* published in 1879 by the Faculty of Science are known as the first research bulletin in Japan. However, such publications then served to report the production of foreign government advisors. It is after 1882 that the achievements of Japanese researchers began to be edited there. It took even more time for other faculties to publish similar bulletins, in fact after the institutional reorganization into the Imperial University of Tokyo. One of the forerunners of such publications was *The Imperial University Bulletin of Medical Science*. The first issue of the bulletin contains famous articles by professors of the Medical University. All text is printed in alphabet on imported paper of the finest quality, and illustrations are lithographed. There are numerous foldout illustrations hand-colored by draftsmen. The present illustration accompanies the text of a research in toxicology on blowfish, written by Juntaro Takahashi (1856 – 1920), then professor of Pharmacology. Takahashi, who studied pharmacology in Berlin and Strasbourg, returned to Japan at the end of October 1885, and was appointed general affairs official at the University of Tokyo the following month, teaching Pharmacology as a full-time lecturer at the Medical University. In Japan, Theodor Eduard Hoffmann (1837 – 1894), Erwin von Bälz (1849 – 1913) and Gentoku Ito (1850 – 1895) had taught Pharmacology alongside Internal Medicine. If we look back at this historical process, we can consider Takahashi's appointment as professor in 1886 as the founding year of the Laboratory of Pharmacology. Takahashi's well-known accomplishments include his research on the physiological action of blowfish poison, led with assistant professor Kichindo Inoko (1866 – 1893). He started his research two years after returning from his overseas study, in 1887. This opened the way for experimental pharmacology based on animal testing. Blowfish poison is present in raw fish, and is easily dissolved in water. From this, Takahashi established that blowfish poison is not a protein, and attempted to draw a "chart of toxicity." The present illustration is laid with gum arabic on the parts representing the fish body, wonderfully reproducing the slime-like texture of the body surface. The superior quality of printing is due to the great authority of the Faculty of Medicine of the Imperial University.

帝國大學紀要

醫科

MITTHEILUNGEN

AUS DER

MEDICINISCHEN FACULTÄT

DER

KAISERLICH-JAPANISCHEN

UNIVERSITÄT.

I Band.

帝國大學印行

明治廿五年

Tokio 1892.

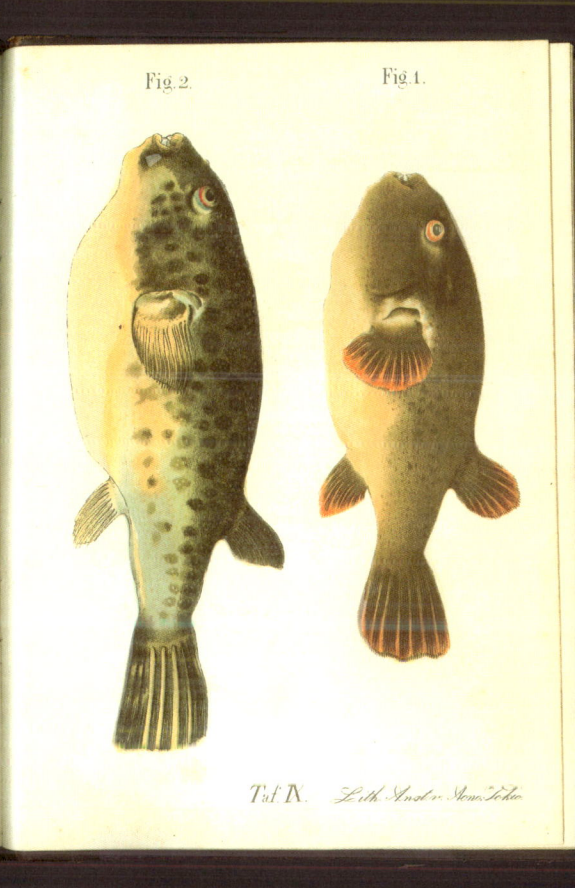

Fig. 2.   Fig. 1.

Taf. IX.   Lith. Anst. v. Stone Tokio

The Miyake Family Collection

   This is the heritage of the Miyake family, whose contribution to the development of modern medicine was considerable. The Miyake house was located in the actual Koishikawa Takehayacho district in Bunkyo ward. The head of the family, Gonsai (1817 – 1868), was a Dutch-style surgeon native of the province of Hizen. His oldest son Hiizu (1848 – 1938), named Mataichi during his childhood, was the youngest attendant to the 1863 delegation to Europe. Upon returning to Japan, he learned English under James Curtis Hepburn (1815 – 1911) in Yokohama. He then studied medicine for two years under the American physician A.M. Vedder, to whom he was introduced by Hepburn. He specialized in pathology, acceding to the status of director of the Tokyo School of Medicine, and eventually making his way to the House of Peers. With his son Koichi (1876 – 1954) in psychiatry and his grandson Masashi (1908 – 1969) in pathology, the family held the position of professor at the Faculty of Medicine of the University of Tokyo over three generations. It thus forms a family of doctors representative of modern Japan, rivaling the Katsuragawa family, known as a clan of doctors at the end of the Edo period. The collection preserved by the Miyake family through the ravages of earthquakes and war includes not only medical and pharmacological specimens, but also natural history specimens covering zoology, botany and mineralogy, as well as medical devices, laboratory instruments, souvenirs, diaries, letters and photographs – amounting to 325 sets including 5000 letters, and totaling more than 10000 items. Historically significant materials are numerous, including among others and in chronological order, the heritage of the householder Gonsai, the items from the 1860 shogunate delegation to America and those from the 1863 shogunate delegation to France.

三宅一族コレクション

　近代医学の発展に多大な貢献のあった三宅一族の遺品である。三宅家は現在の文京区小石川竹早町にあった。肥前出身の家長良齋(1817–1868)は外科の蘭方医であった。長男の幼名「復一」、後の秀(1848–1938)は、文久3(1863)年遣欧使節団に最年少の随員として加わり、帰国後、横浜でジェームス・カーティス・ヘボン(1815–1911)について英語を学んでいる。さらにヘボンに紹介された米国人医師A.M.ヴェッダーの許で2年間に亘って医学を修め、病理学の医家となり、やがて東京医学校校長心得を皮切りに、最終的に貴族院議員まで出世街道を上り詰めた。その息子の鑛一(1876–1954)の精神病学、さらには孫の仁(1908–1969)の病理学と、三代に亘って東京大学医学部教授の任を負っている。江戸後期に医家一門として知られた桂川家にも比肩し得る、近代日本の医家一族だったのである。三宅一族が、震災、戦災から守り抜いたコレクションは、医学や薬学はもとより、動物・植物・鉱物の自然史標本類、医療器具、実験道具、記念品、日記、書簡、写真など、件数にして325件、書簡だけでも5千点に上り、総数にして1万点を優に超える。来歴別に言うと、家長良齋の遺品、万延元(1860)年幕府遣外(遣米)使節団将来品、文久3(1863)年の幕府遣欧(遣仏)使節団将来品など、歴史的に見て重要な資料が多数含まれている。

036

天秤
江戸時代／金属、ガラス、木製台、木製箱入り／本体長235、皿直径70、箱縦135、横275、高50／東京大学総合研究博物館所蔵 三宅コレクション

小型で携行に便利な天秤ばかりである。日本人は古くから、小型で、可愛らしいものを作るのを得意としてきた。ここにもそのモノ作り精神の何たるかが顕れている。

Balance
Edo period / Metal, glass, wooden base, in wooden case / Balance: L235, D70; Case: L275, W135, H50 / Miyake collection, UMUT

A small, portable balance. Since old times, the Japanese are good at making small-scale, pretty objects. Such spirit for conceiving objects can also be seen here.

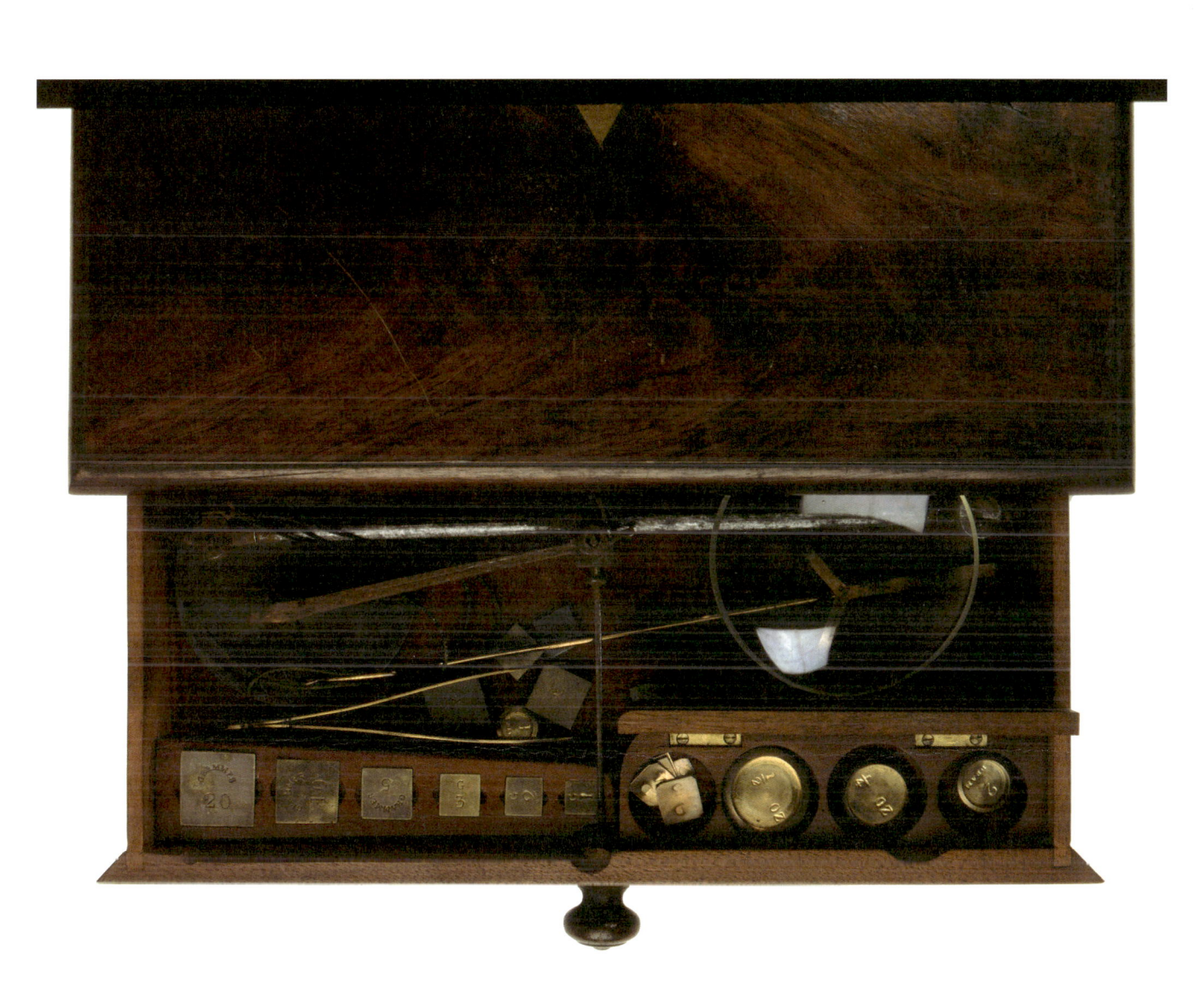

038

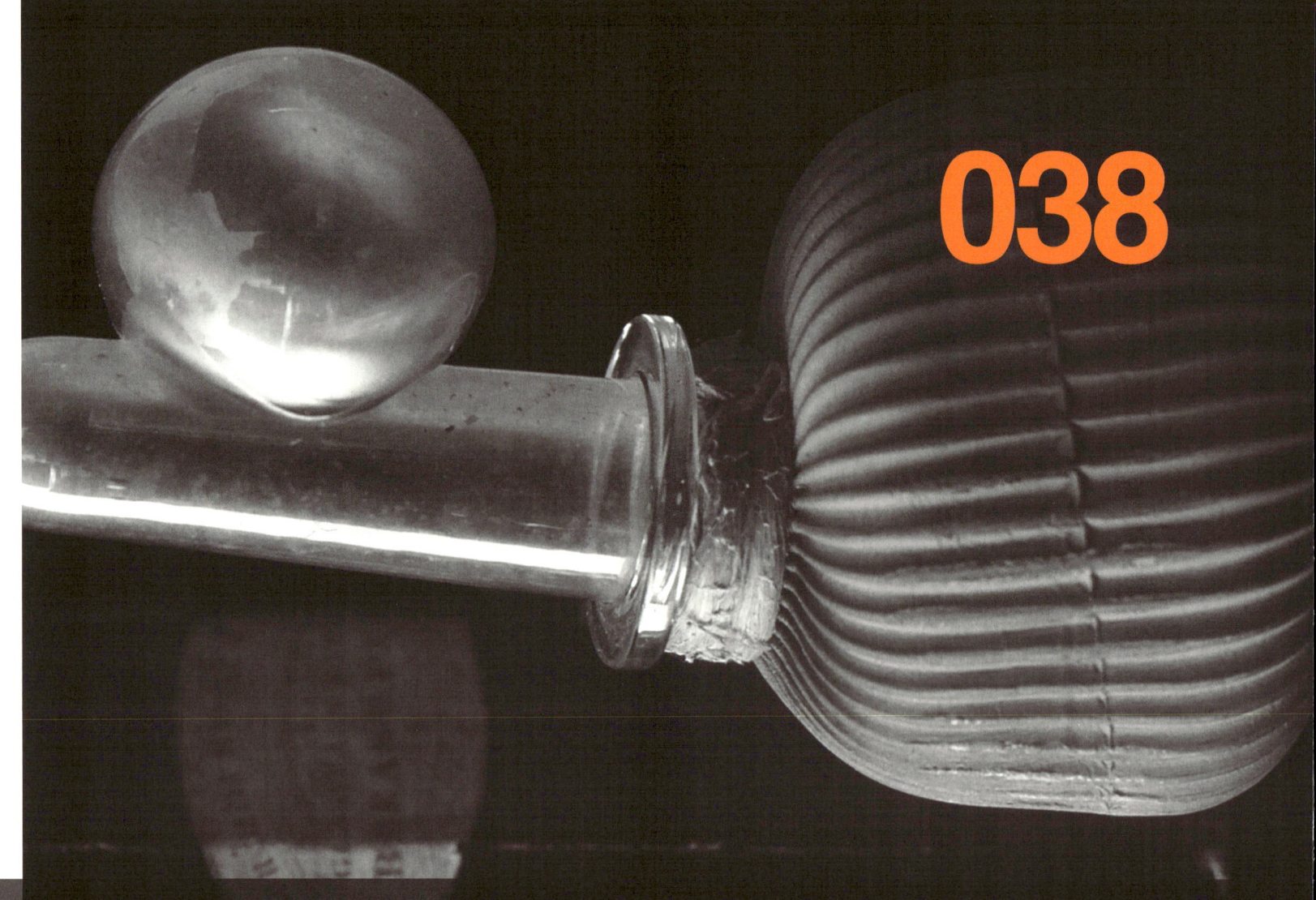

搾乳器
弘化5（1848）年以降／ユニオン天然ゴム有限会社製／ガラス、ゴム、紙製箱付き／高200、箱底幅90、箱高220／東京大学総合研究博物館所蔵三宅コレクション

本体に「UNION INDIA RUBBER Co / GOODYEAR'S PATENT / NEW YORK / 1844 & 48」の刻字あり。箱ラベルには「Union India Rubber Company / Exclusive Manufacturer / GOODYEAR'S PATENT / BREAST PUMP / NEW YORK」とある。三宅一族の家長艮齋（1817–1868）の遺品であるとすると、万延元（1860）年幕府遣外（遣米）使節団の将来品の可能性もある。さもなくば、三宅秀（1848–1938）が東京医学校の教官筆頭として、校長長與専齋（1838–1902）に随い、明治9（1876）年の米国フィラデルフィア市万国医学会に出席したさいに、米国で購入したものであろう。1844年と48年にニューヨークで特許を取得した製品である。天然ゴムで作られた搾乳器が、当時としては珍しいものだったということである。

Milking Machine
After 1848 / Made by Union India Rubber Co. / Glass, rubber, with paper box / H200; Box: W90, H220 / Miyake collection, UMUT

Bears the engraving "Union India Rubber Co/Goodyear's Patent/New York/1844&48." "Union India Rubber Company/Exclusive Manufacturer/Goodyear's Patent/Breast Pump/New York" printed on the box. If we consider that it was left by Gonsai (1817 – 1868), head of the Miyake family, this item may come from the 1860 shogunate delegation to America. Otherwise, it may have been bought by Hiizu (1848 – 1938) in the United States when, as the chief instructor of the Tokyo School of Medicine, he followed the school director Sensai Nagayo (1838 – 1902) to attend the 1876 International Medical Convention in Philadelphia. This product was patented in 1844 and 1848 in New York, implying that a milking machine made of natural rubber was a rare item at the time.

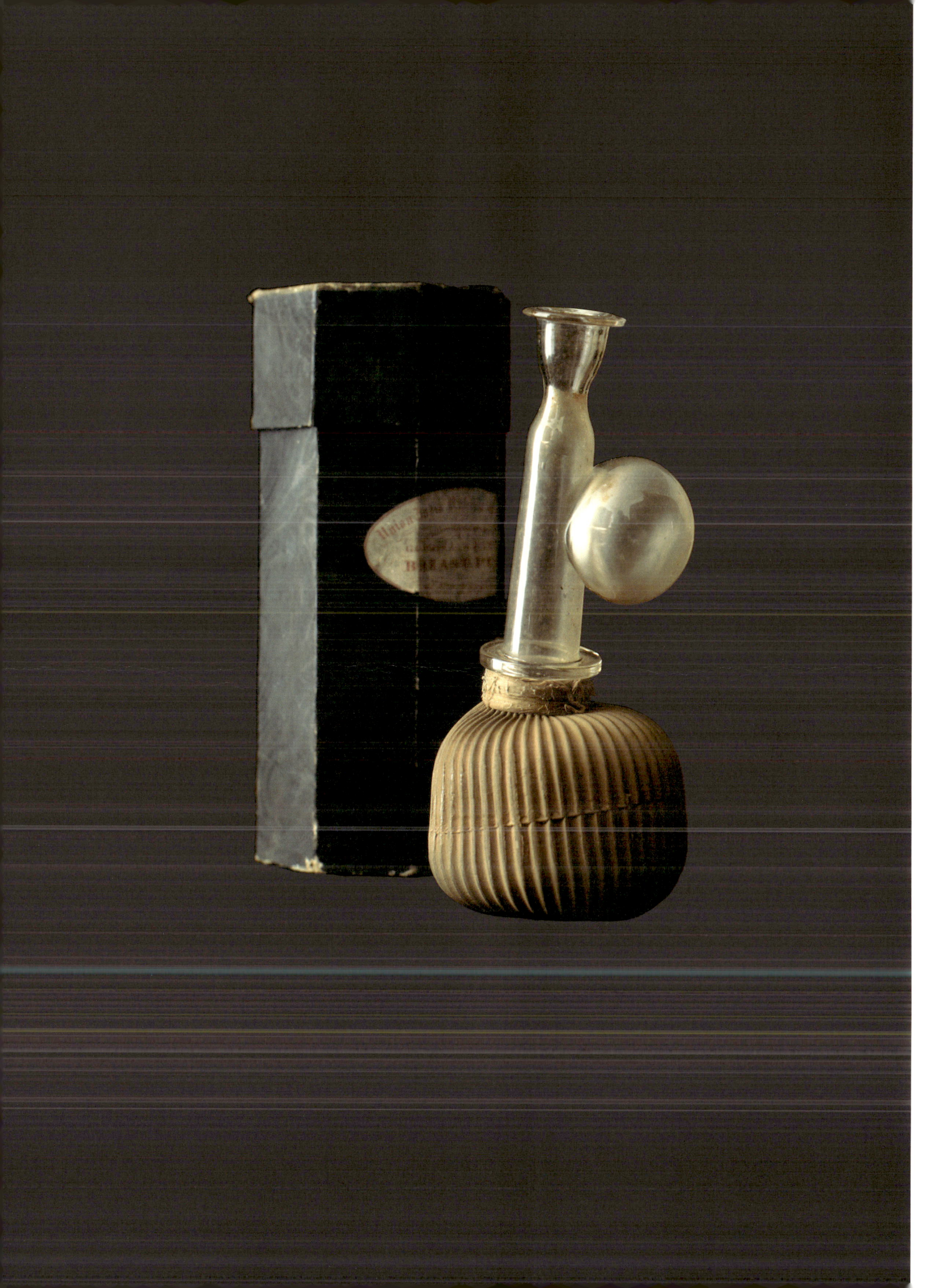

040

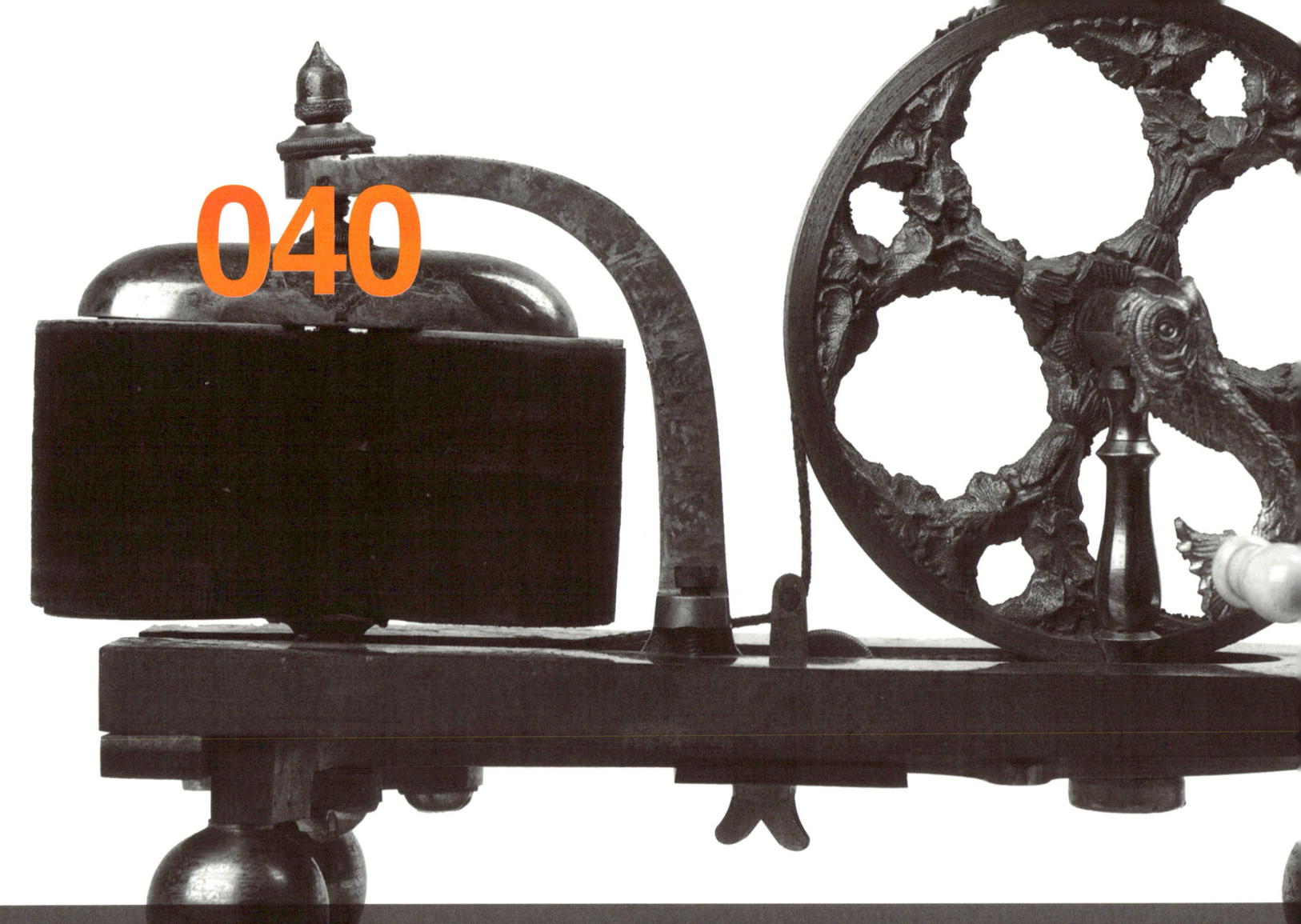

医療用電気器

文久3(1863)年以前／金属製滑車・錨、鉄製台座、象牙製柄、糸、貝、ビロード、木製箱入り／本体長84、幅204、高150、箱縦246、横170、高105／東京大学総合研究博物館所蔵三宅コレクション

箱蓋内側に「文久三年　千八百六十三年ニ巴里ニテ購入シタル医療用電気器」との付箋が貼付されており、三宅秀(1848−1938)が文久3(1863)年の幕府遣欧使節団に随行したさいに、パリで購入したことがわかる。

Electric Medical Equipment

Before 1863 / Pulley and anchor in metal, iron base, ivory handle, thread, shell, velvet, in wooden box / Mechanism: L84, W204, H150; Box: L246, W170, H105 / Miyake collection, UMUT

A tag bearing the mention in Japanese "Electric medical equipment bought in Paris in the third year of Bunkyu, in 1863" is glued in the inner part of the lid, indicating that this was bought by Hiizu Miyake (1848 – 1938) in Paris when he followed the 1863 shogunate delegation to Europe.

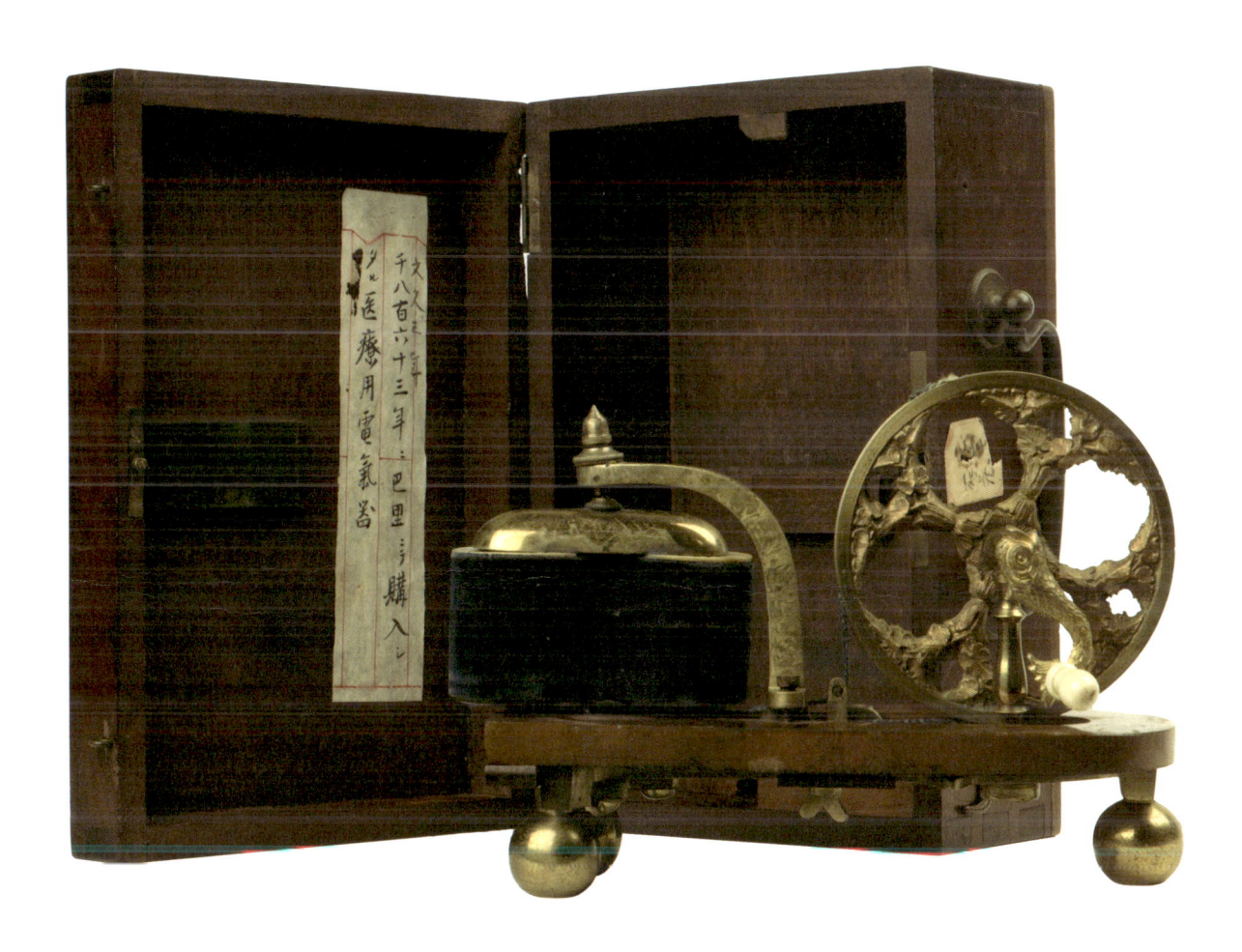

大久保家旧蔵
千八百六十三年ニ巴里ニテ購入ス
医療用電気器

042

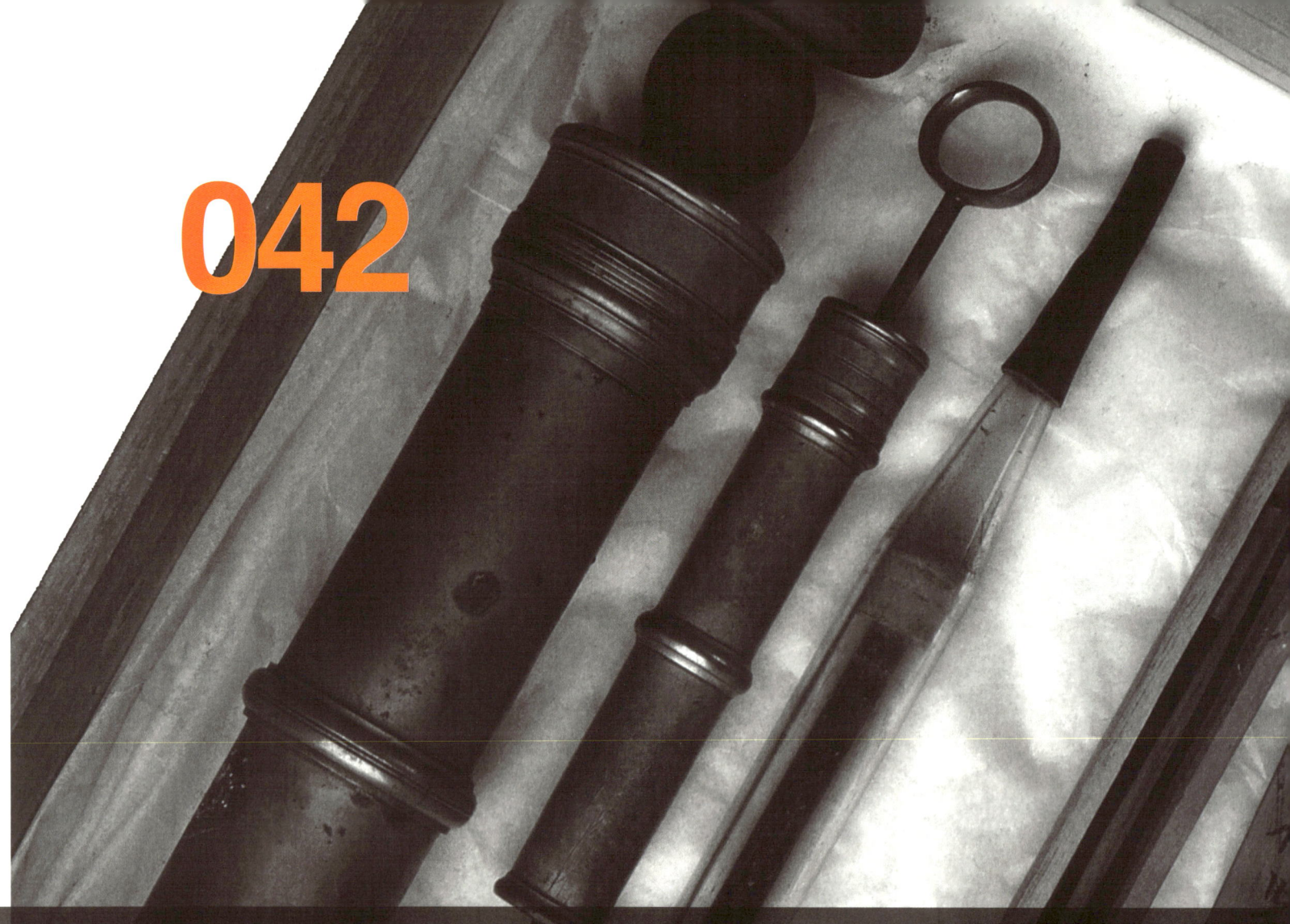

外科道具セット
文久3(1863)年以前／マチュー商会製他／金属、木製三段重箱入り／外箱縦285、横395、高230／東京大学総合研究博物館所蔵三宅コレクション

メス1点(刻字「LEITER」)、ハサミ1点、ピンセット1点、鉗子2点、「探丸器」13点、消息子7点、カテーテル1点、腹鏡1点、注射針2点、ゴム片1点、シリンジ3点、聴診器1点、補聴器2点、止血帯4点、脱腸帯1点、糸3点、紐1点、綿1点、紙1点(筒ラベル「PAPIER FAYARD ET BLAYN」)が収められている。三宅復一(秀)(1848–1938)の残した『航海日記』の4月5日のくだりには、「二時ヨリ博物館ニ至リ、又外科道具ヤニ至リ、少シ許リ道具ヲ買フ」とあり、さらに4月27日のそれには「外科道具屋ニ至リ種々ノ外科道具ヲ買(見)タリ」とある。ここに言う「外科道具屋」とは、パリ市内ラテン区の医学部通りのすぐわき、ランシエンヌ・コメディ街28番地に店舗を構えていた外科道具製造業マチュー商会のことを指している。そのことは三宅の手許に残されていた1864年版販売目録から判る。三宅コレクションのなかに残されているフランス製医療器具の多くは、おそらく上記の商店で購われたものであろう。

Set of Surgical Instruments
Before 1863 / Made by L. Mathieu Co. / Metal, in 3-layered wooden box / Outer box: L285, W395, H230 / Miyake collection, UMUT

Contains a scalpel (with the engraving "Leiter"), a pair of scissors, a pair of tweezers, 2 forceps, 13 bullet removal tools, 7 probes, a catheter, a laparoscope, 2 hypodermic needles, a piece of rubber, 3 syringes, a sthethoscope, 2 hearing aids, 4 tourniquets, a hernia belt, 3 pieces of thread, a string, a piece of cotton and a piece of paper (a cylindrical "Papier Fayard et Blayn" label). Mataichi (Hiizu) Miyake (1848 – 1938) held a *Navigation Journal,* in which we find written, dated April 5: "From two o'clock, went at the museum, then went again at the surgical instrument shop, and bought a few instruments." Dated April 27, we find: "Went at the surgical instrument shop and bought (saw) a few surgical instruments." The "surgical instrument shop" mentioned here is Mathieu, located on 28 rue de l'Ancienne Comédie, near the rue de l'Ecole de Médecine in the Latin Quarter of Paris. The shop sold the products of the Mathieu company, manufacturer of surgical instruments. This is attested by the 1864 sales catalogue left among Miyake's possessions. Most of the French-made medical instruments left in the Miyake collection were probably acquired at the abovementioned shop.

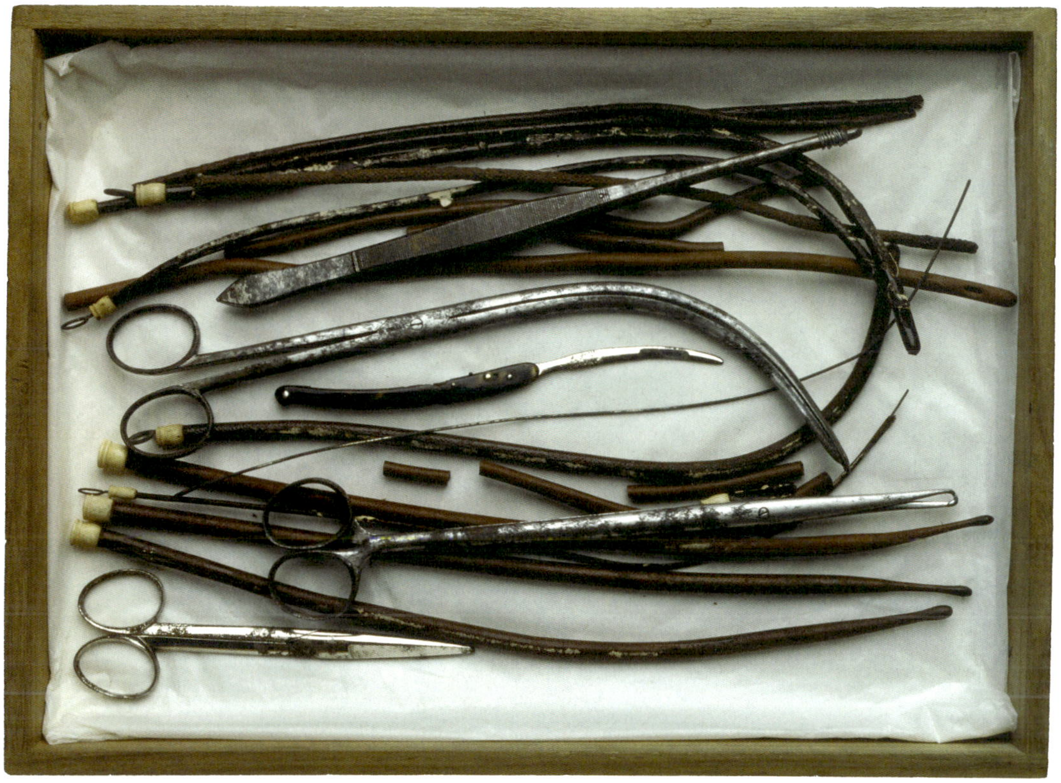

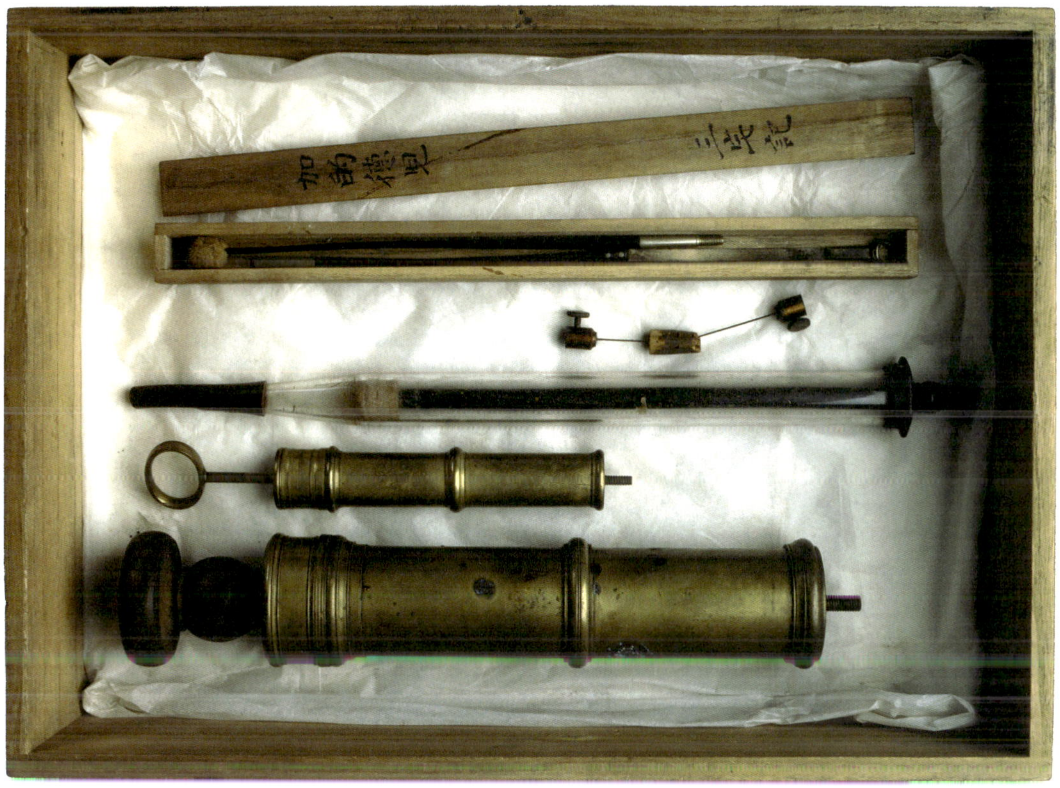

044

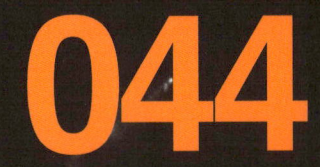

外科道具セット
文久3(1863)年以前／マチュー商会製他／金属、木、鼈甲、木製7段重箱入り／箱縦304、横169、高56、外箱縦322、横187、高295／東京大学総合研究博物館所蔵三宅コレクション

鼈甲製鞘入メス30点、木製柄のメス7点、金属製柄のメス3点、鞘のみ1点、ハサミ4点、ピンセット2点、鉗子5点、消息子2点、針3点、鉤12点、導子3点、カテーテル8点、套管針6点、創縁クリップ1点(箱上書「マチユー造セルファン　一八六三年」)、シリンジ5点、匙5点、針容器2点、糸1点(ラベル「100YARDS / MOLENDINAR WORKS GLASGOW」)、ガラス皿1点、ガラス片2点、部品1点が収められている。一部のハサミ、メス等は鉄砲鍛冶猪俣某作か。

Set of Surgical Instruments
Before 1863 / Made by L. Mathieu Co. / Metal, wood, tortoiseshell, in 7-layered wooden box / Box: L304, W169, H56; Outer box: L322, W187, H295 / Miyake collection, UMUT

Contains 30 tortoiseshell sheath scalpels, 7 scalpels with wooden handle, 3 scalpels with metallic handle, a sheath, 4 scissors, 2 tweezers, 5 forceps, 2 probes, 3 needles, 12 hooks, 3 electrodes, 8 catheters, 6 trocars, a suture clip ("made by Mathieu [...] 1863" written in Japanese on box), 5 syringes, 5 spoons, 2 needle containers, a piece of thread (with the label "100 yards/Molendinar Works Glasgow"), a glass dish, 2 pieces of glass and a component. Some scissors and scalpels may have been made by a certain Inomata, a blacksmith producing guns.

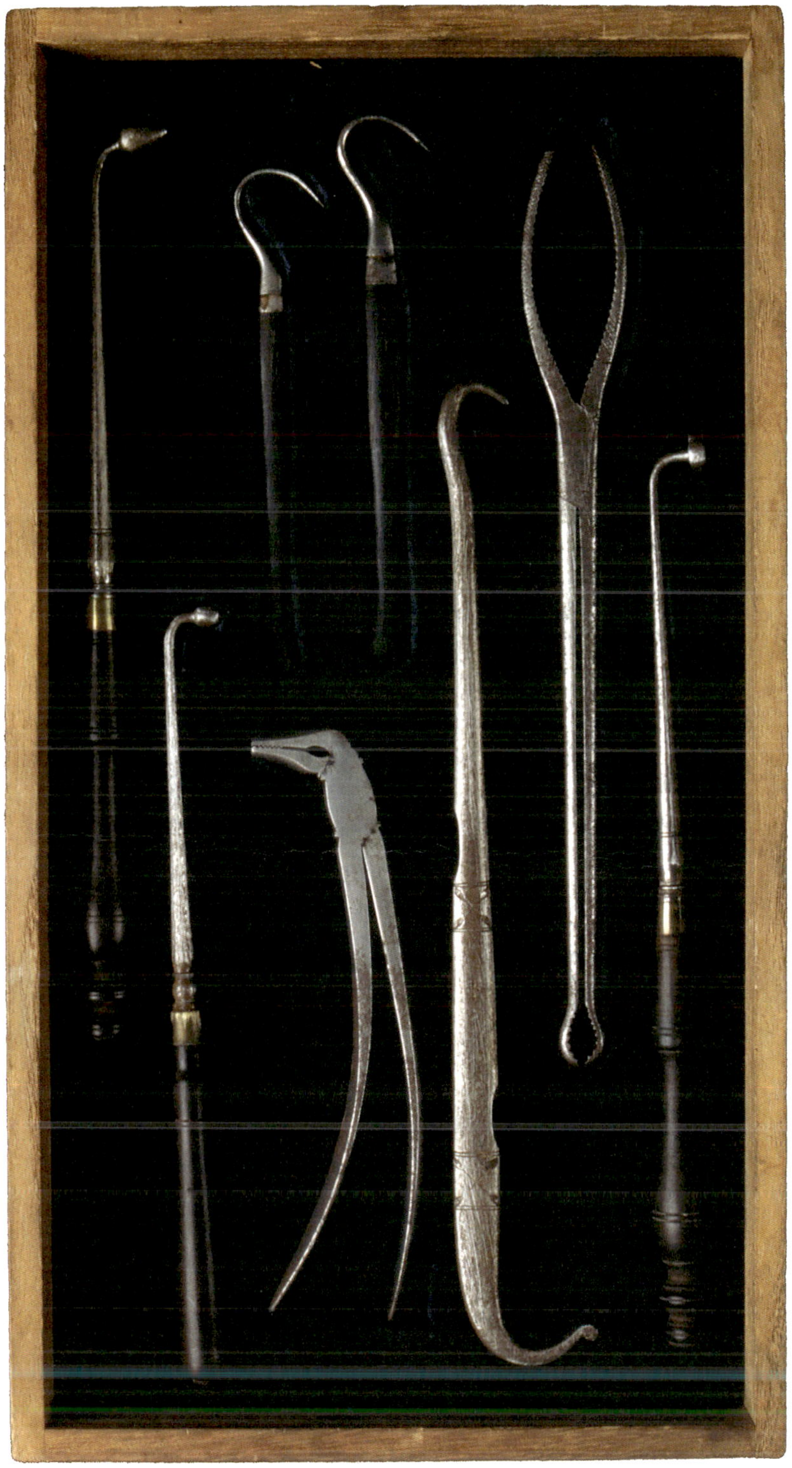

046

注射筒（シリンジ）
年代未詳／金属、木製箱／本体長200、箱長255、幅145、高50／東京大学総合研究博物館所蔵三宅コレクション

Syringe
Date unknown / Metal, wooden box / Syringe: L200; Box: L255, W145, H50 / Miyake collection, UMUT

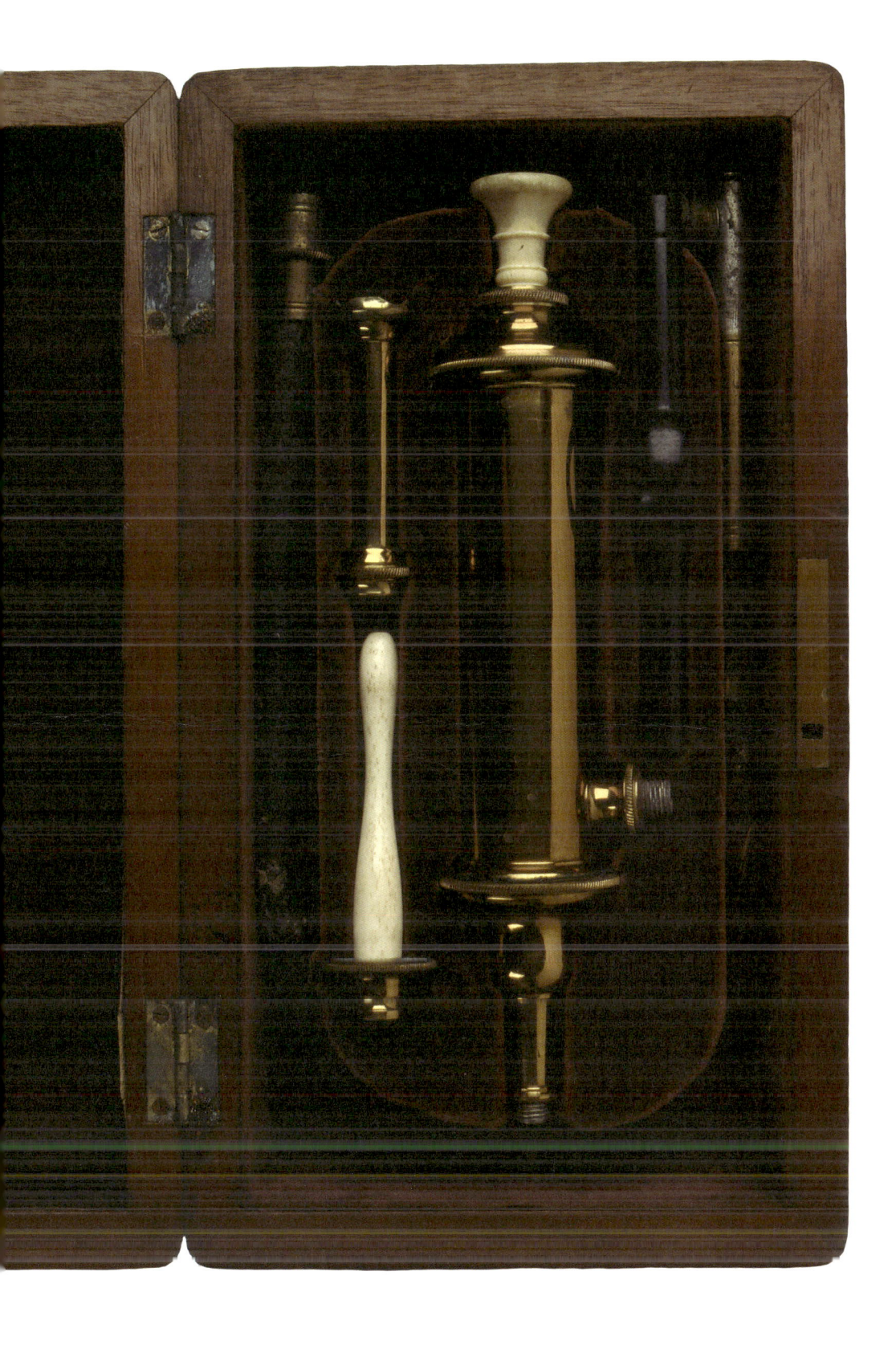

048

眼病標本
明治17(1884)年頃／トラモン商会／蝋細工、顔料、ガラス、木製箱入り／標本長65、幅68、箱縦95、横125、高52／東京大学総合研究博物館所蔵三宅コレクション

眼病の症例を示す蝋細工標本である。蝋細工の技術を完成させたのは17世紀のイタリア人ガエターノ・ジューリオ・ズンボ(1656–1701)である。ボローニャの神父であったズンボは、その技術の高さを伝え聞いたルイ14世の要請を受け、1701年5月にフランスの科学アカデミーでイタリアから持参した蝋製人頭解剖模型を供覧している。パリ大学の解剖学博物館にはそのときの記念すべき標本が保存されている。以来、18世紀のフランスでは医学標本の多くに蝋細工技術が用いられることになった。19世紀半ばになると、解剖学者ルイ・マリウス・フェラトン(1797–1880)の指導で蝋製医学標本が技術的な完成をみることになった。世紀後半にはパリの医学部通りにそれを専業とするトラモン商会が開業し、この専門店はパリの万国博覧会にも蝋細工標本を出品している。本標本には、保護材として、パリで1884年初頭に発行された日刊紙『ラ・フランス』(巻号不明)が使われている。付帯する仏語新聞の存在は、三宅秀(1848–1938)が2度目の渡仏のさいにトラモン商会で標本を購入したと考える状況証拠となる。瞳が青いのも、西洋で制作されたことの証である。

Eye Disease Specimen
Circa 1884 / Made by Maison Tramond / Wax, pigment, glass, in wooden box / Specimen: L65, W68; Box: L125, W95, H52 / Miyake collection, UMUT

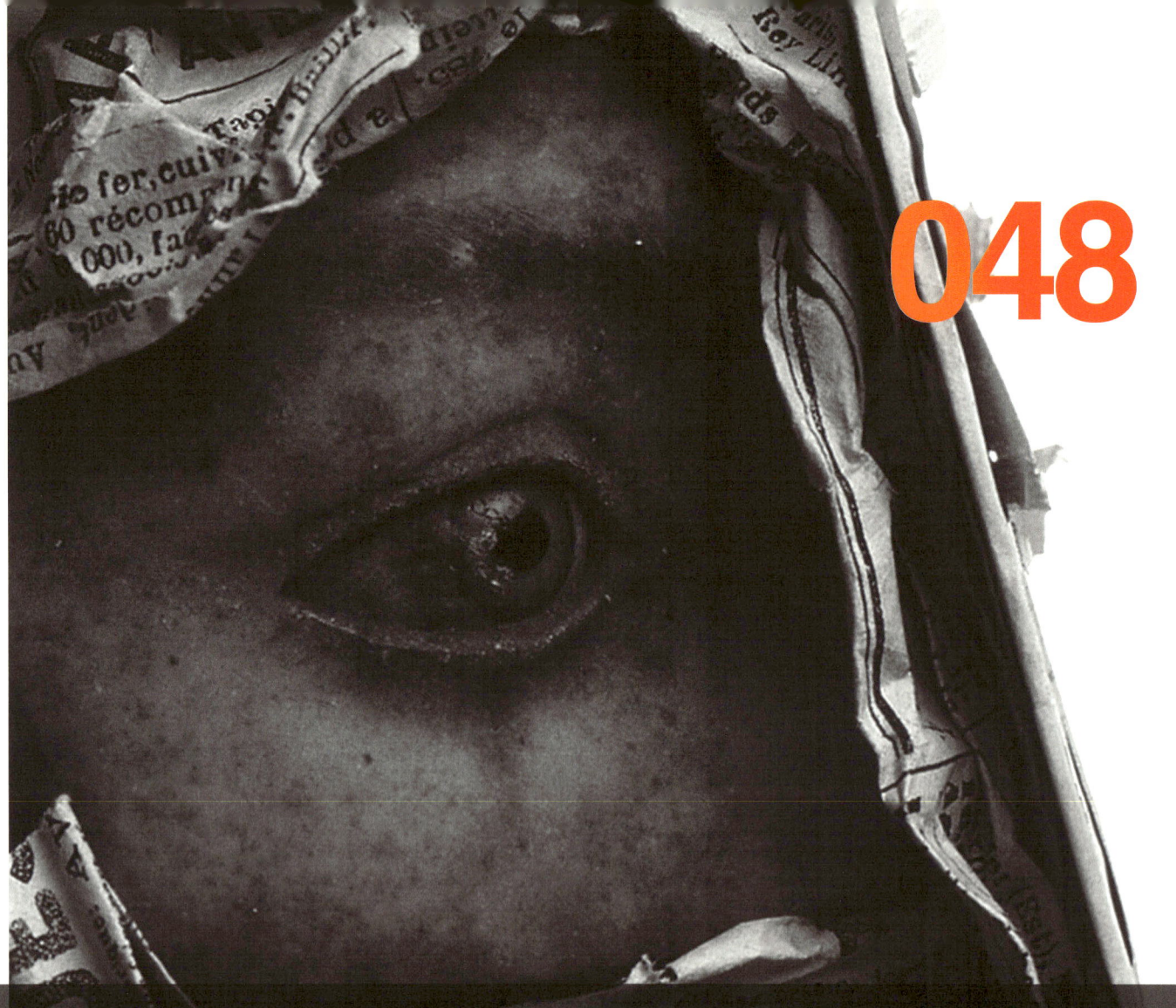

Wax specimen representing the symptoms of an eye disease. It is Gaetano Giulio Zumbo (1656 – 1701) who, in 17th-Century Italy, developed the technique of wax modeling. Word of Zumbo, who was an abbot in Bologna, and of his high technique eventually went to Louis XIV, and upon the latter's demand, he presented in May 1701 to the French Science Academy a wax model of a human head he had brought from Italy. This memorable specimen is now preserved at the Museum of Anatomy of the University of Paris. Thereafter, wax modeling was commonly used in 18th-Century France for medical specimens. In mid 19th Century, under the impulsion of Louis-Marius Ferraton (1797 – 1880), the technique of wax modeling for medical specimens was perfected. The Maison Tramond, specialized in this technique, opened in the rue de l'Ecole de Médecine in Paris in the second half of the 19th Century, and exhibited wax specimens at the Universal Exposition. The present specimen is wrapped with a sheet of the daily newspaper *La France* (date unknown) published in Paris in the beginning of 1884. This proves that the specimen was acquired at the Maison Tramond by Hiizu Miyake (1848 – 1938) during his second stay in France. The blue color of the pupil testifies that the specimen was made in the West.

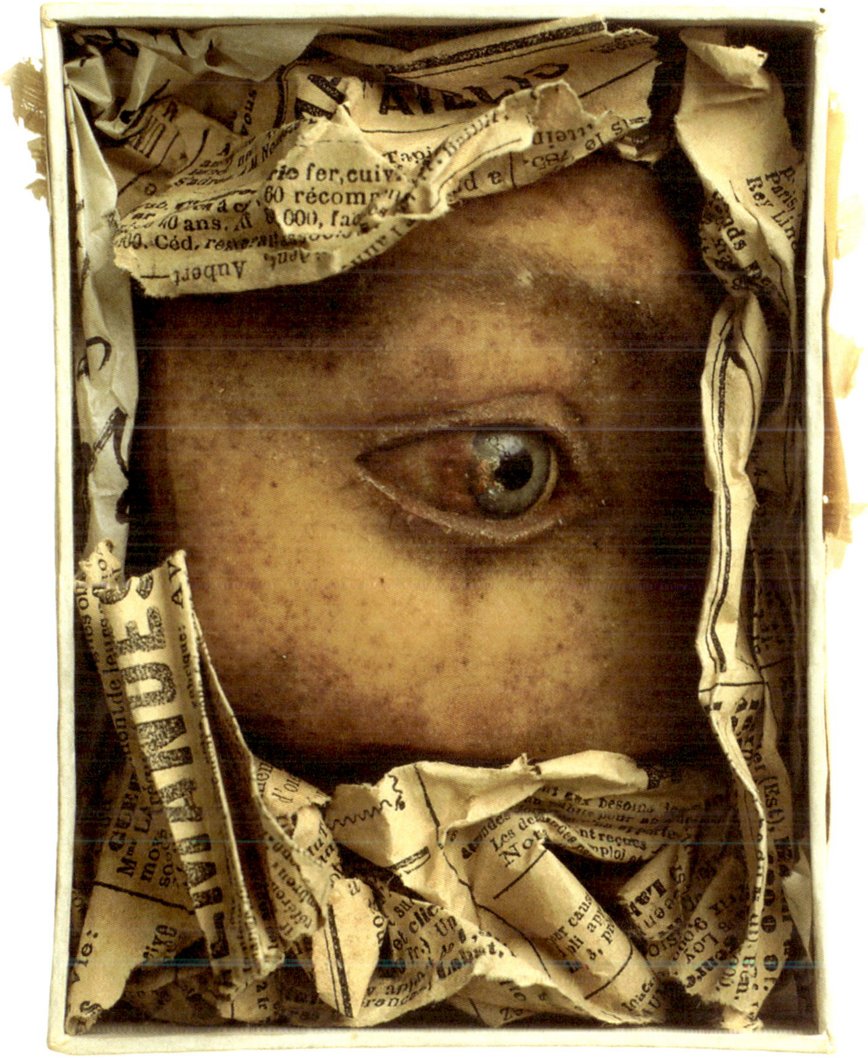

050

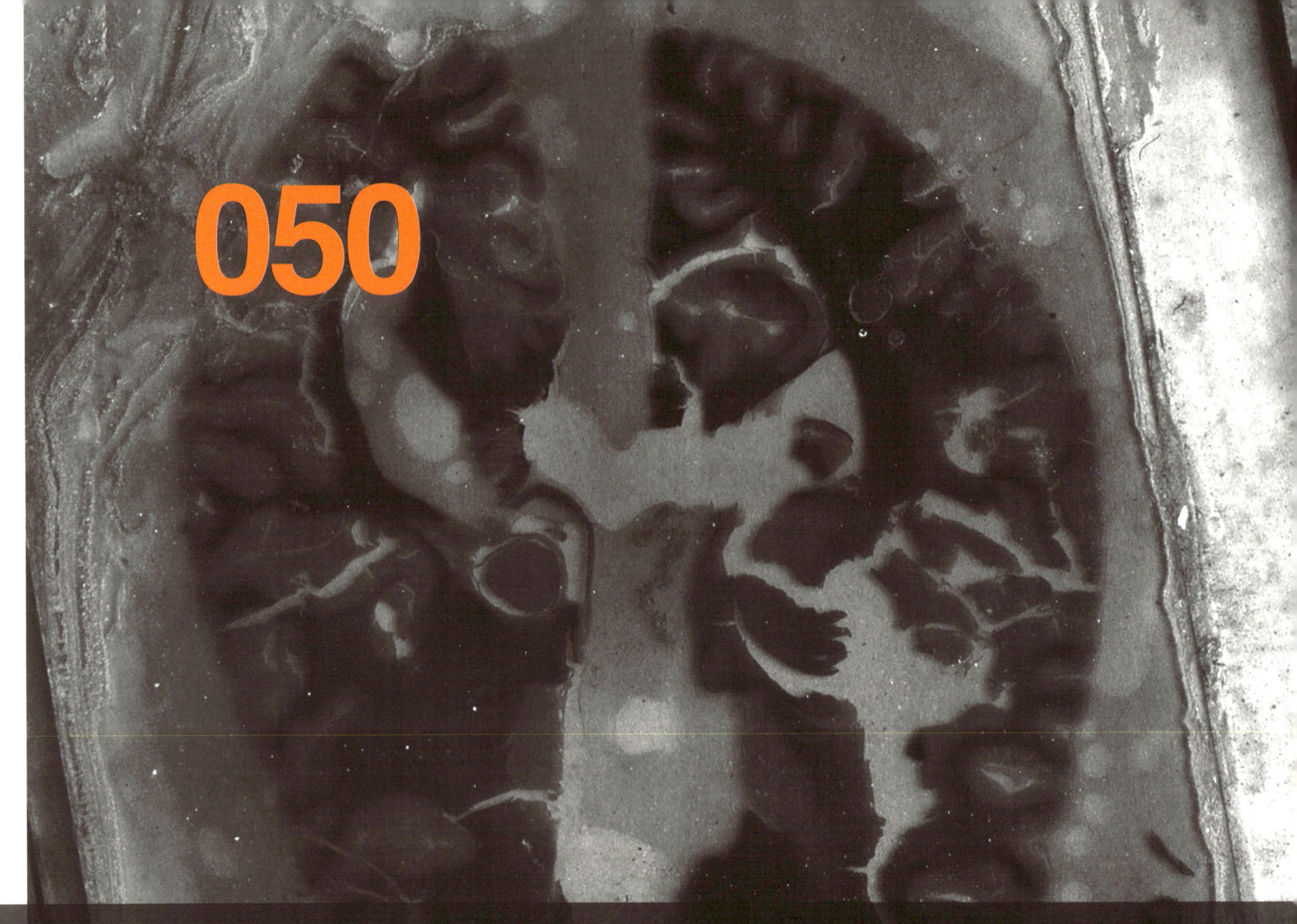

脳切片プレパラート標本
年代未詳／プレパラート、カバーガラス、厚紙台紙貼り／台紙縦242、横184／東京大学総合研究博物館所蔵 三宅コレクション

切片プレパラートは生体の有力な保存法のひとつである。現代では生体にシリコンを充填させて作るプラスティネーションが医学標本の主流となっている。

Brain Slice Specimen for Microscope
Date unknown / Slice, glass, glued on cardboard / Cardboard: L242, W184 / Miyake collection, UMUT

Slices are an efficient method of conservation of living organisms. Currently, plastination, which consists in injecting silicon in the organism, is the main method for making medical specimens.

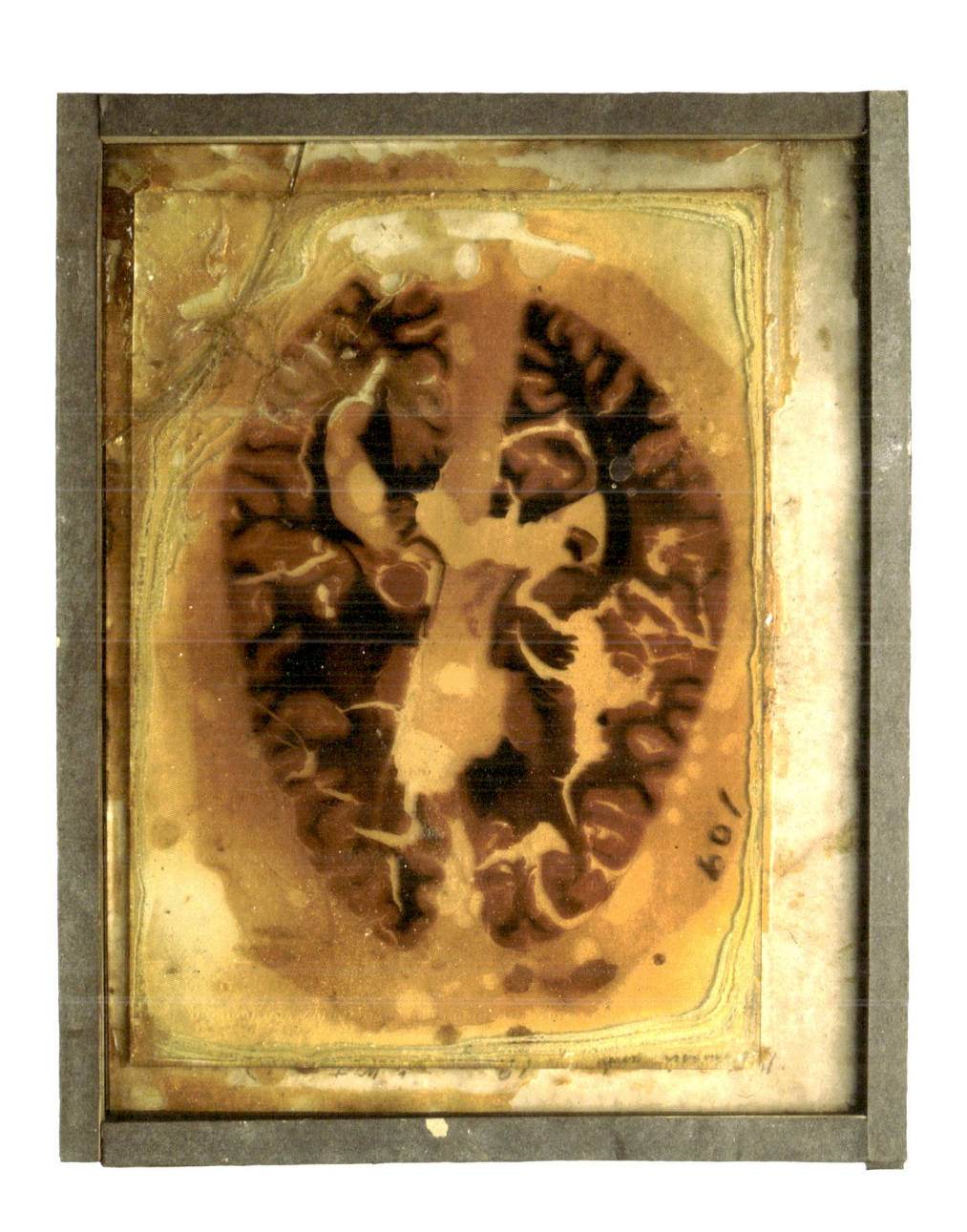

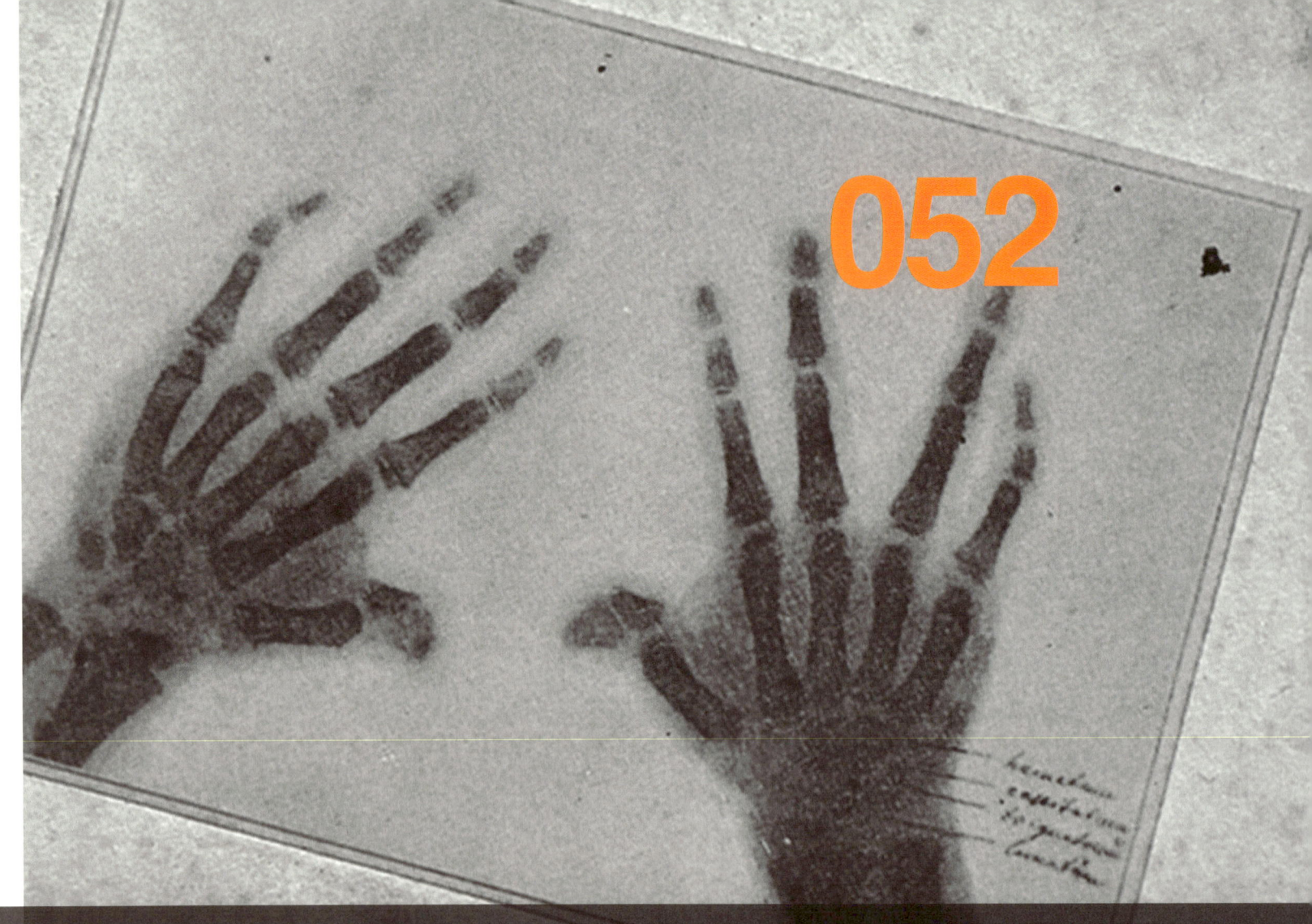

手のレントゲン写真

明治33(1900)年前後／レントゲン写真、印画紙焼き、厚紙台紙貼り／本紙縦55、横80、台紙縦130、横190／東京大学医学部精神病学教室旧蔵／総合研究博物館所蔵三宅コレクション

帝大医科大学解剖学教室にエックス線装置が導入されたのは、明治30(1897)年のことである。翌年には病院に、2年後には内科にもそれが設置された。明治14(1881)年に来日し、眼科、婦人科、皮膚科の講義を担当したドイツ人教師ユリウス・カール・スクリバ(1848-1905)もまた、明治34(1901)年帝大での任期を終えて一時帰国したさい、同様の装置をドイツから運び帰り、それは外科に設置された。明治30(1897)年3月17日にスクリバは東京医学会で「人体透視」を供覧している。

Radiograph of a Hand

Circa 1900 / Radiograph on photographic paper, mounted on cardboard / Photograph: L55, W80; Cardboard: L130, W190 / Former collection of the Laboratory of Psychiatry, Faculty of Medicine, The University of Tokyo / Miyake collection, UMUT

The X-ray device was introduced in the Laboratory of Anatomy of the Imperial Medical University in 1897. It was then set up within the hospital the following year, and at the Internal Medicine Department two years after. Julius Karl Scriba (1848 – 1905), who arrived in Japan in 1881 and taught ophthalmology, gynecology and dermatology, and who once returned home in 1901 upon the expiration of his term at the Imperial University, brought back such a device from Germany, which was set up at the External Medicine Department. On March 17 1897, Scriba presented the "perspective on the human body" at the Tokyo Medical Conference.

精神病學敎室

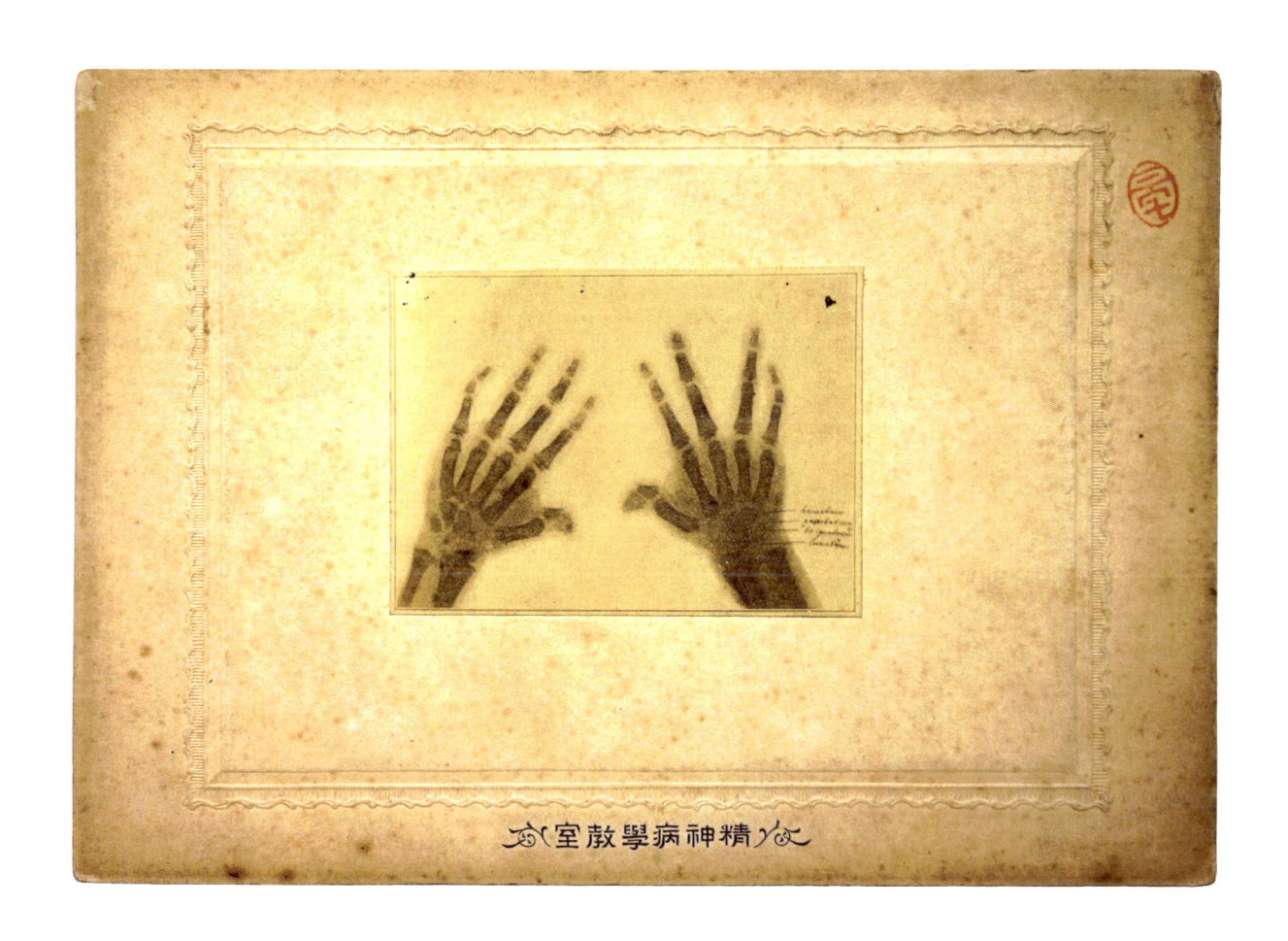

054

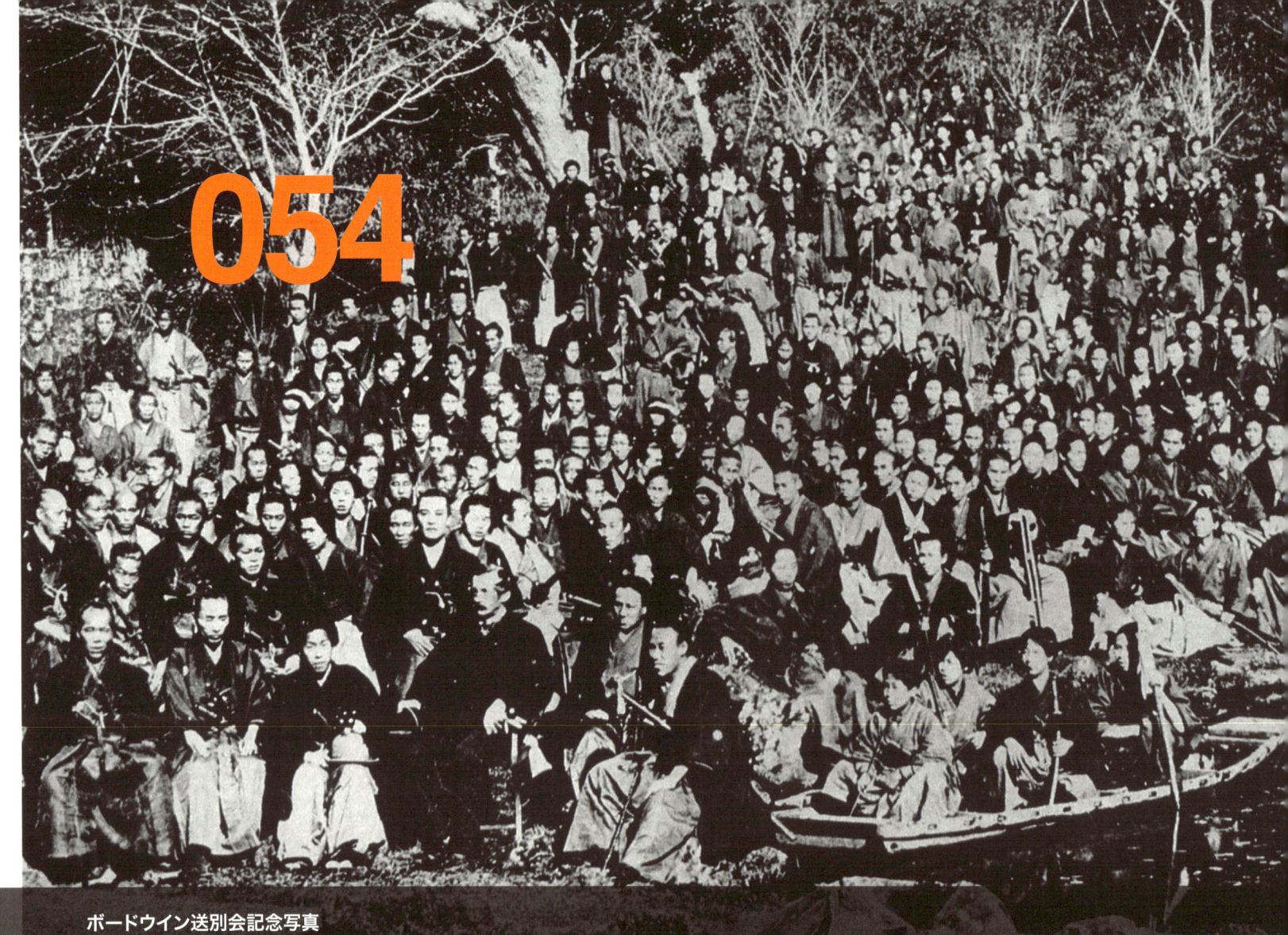

ボードウイン送別会記念写真
明治3(1870)年閏10月／撮影者未詳／鶏卵紙写真／縦209, 横277／東京大学総合研究博物館所蔵三宅コレクション

写真裏に「大学東校御雇外人教師ボードウィン氏送別会記念写真」の貼紙あり。幕府がオランダ人軍医ポンペ・ファン・メールデルフォールト(1829–1907)の後任として文久2(1862)年に招聘したのが、オランダ陸軍一等軍医のアントニウス・フランシスカス・ボードウィン(1820–1885)であった。長崎養生所頭取となったボードウィンは、江戸にオランダ系軍医学校・理学校を創設するよう幕府に進言している。その準備のため慶應3(1866)年に緒方惟準(1843–1909)ら留学生を伴って一時帰国を果たしたボードウィンは、翌年再来日するが、幕府は瓦解し、明治新政府がドイツ式医学の導入に路線変更したことで、明治3(1870)年6月、オランダ式医学校建設計画を実現せぬまま帰国することになった。しかし、普仏戦争の煽りを受け、後任のドイツ人医師の来日が遅れたため、ボードウィンは東校での講義を続け、帰国が10月まで延期された。新政府はボードウィンの功績に報いるべく金3千両を贈り、併せて小石川薬園で盛大な送別会を開催している。写真はそのときに撮影されたものと思われる。

Commemorative Photograph of Bauduin's Farewell Reception
October 1870 / Photographer unknown / Photograph on albumen paper / L209, W277 / Miyake collection, UMUT

The notice, written in Japanese, "Commemorative photograph of the Farewell Reception of Bauduin, Foreign government advisor to the Eastern College" is glued on the back of the photograph. Anthonius Franciscus Bauduin (1820 – 1885), first-class medical officer of the Dutch Army, was invited by the shogunate in 1862 as the successor to Dutch medical officer Pompe van Meerdervoort (1829 – 1907). Named director of the Nagasaki Hospital, Bauduin advised the shogunate to establish a Dutch-style military school of medicine and science. Bauduin, who once returned home in 1866 for that purpose, taking along with him students such as Ijun Ogata (1843 – 1909), came back to Japan the following year. However, with the collapse of the shogunate and the adoption of German medicine by the new Meiji government, he resigned to return home in June 1870 without having realized his plans to build a Dutch-style medicine school. But his German successor's arrival in Japan was retarded by the Franco-Prussian War, and Bauduin continued his teaching at the Eastern College, his return having been postponed to October. The new government, acknowledging Bauduin's contribution, offered him 3000 *ryo* in gold and held a magnificent farewell banquet in the Koishikawa Gardens. The photograph was apparently shot then.

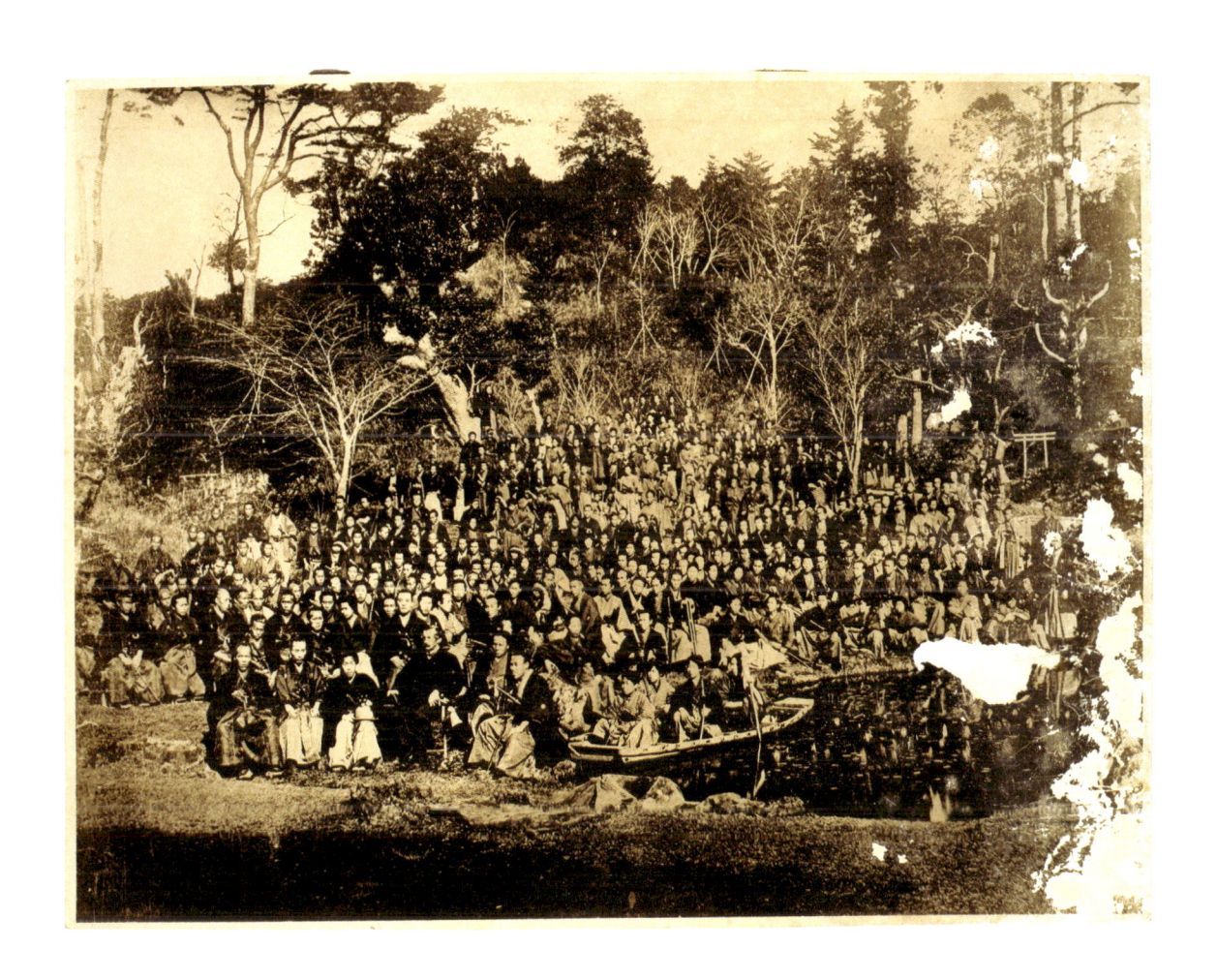

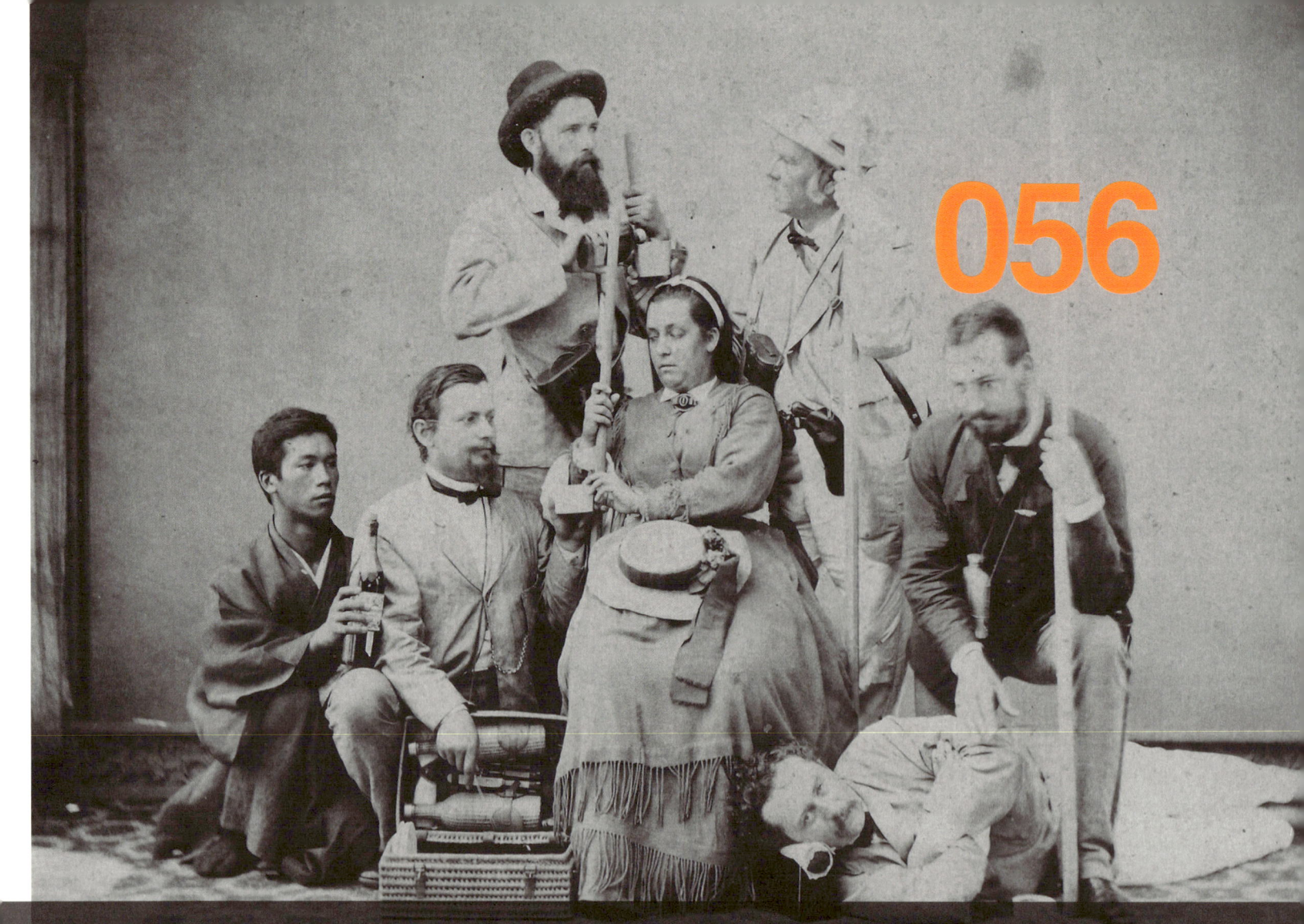

ミュルレル夫妻ほか写真
明治4(1871)年から明治8(1875)年のあいだ／撮影者未詳／鶏卵紙写真、厚紙台紙貼り／本紙縦185、横225、台紙縦285、横355／東京大学総合研究博物館所蔵三宅コレクション

台紙表に墨書で「平臥スルハ　コッヒュース氏／右ニ立テルハ　ミュルレル先生／中ニ坐スルハ同士夫人／傍ニ踞スルハ　フンク氏」と記されている。レオポルト・ミュルレル(1824–1893)はドイツの陸軍軍医。ミュルレルはボン大学とベルリン大学に学び、フリードリッヒ・ヴィルヘルム軍医学校で教官を務めたのち、普仏戦争のさいに野戦病院長と活躍し、その功績が認められ陸軍少佐の地位にあった。明治4(1871)年8月、47歳のときに明治政府の招聘で来日し、東校に着任。同時に着任した海軍軍医で内科医のテオドール・ホフマン(1837–1894)とともに、それまで大学東校で行われてきたオランダ式医学教育に代わり、ドイツ式医学の普及を推進し、東校の教育改革に寄与した。東校に製薬学科を創設し、医薬分業の実現のため薬学教育の定着に努力したのもミュルレルであった。明治5(1872)年3月、明治天皇の東校への行幸が実現し、8月3日新しい学制が施行され、東校は第一大学区医学校と改名された。ミュルレルは雇用契約を満了したのち、明治8(1875)年11月、帰国の途に就いている。写真は御雇い外国人教師たちの余興を捉えたもので、コッヒュースは理化学と数学、フンクはドイツ語とラテン語を講じた。

Photograph of the Muller Couple and Others
Between 1871 and 1875 / Photographer unknown / Photograph on albumen paper, mounted on cardboard / Photograph: L185, W225; Cardboard: L285, W355 / Miyake collection, UMUT

On the back of the cardboard, the names of the persons appearing on the picture are written in ink in Japanese. Benjamin Carl Leopold Muller (1824 – 1893) was a German medical officer. He studied at the University of Bonn and at the University of Berlin before teaching at the Friedrich Wilhelm Military School of Medicine. He served as director of a field hospital during the Franco-Prussian War, and was named major of the Army in recognition of his contribution. In August 1871 at the age of 47, he came to Japan invited by the Meiji government, and took up his post at the Eastern College. Along with the Navy medical officer and doctor of internal medicine Theodor Eduard Hoffmann (1837 – 1894), who started working at the same time, he promoted the spread of German medicine in replacement of the Dutch medical education that had been conducted until then at the Eastern College, contributing to its educational reform. It was also Muller who created the Department of Pharmaceutics at the Eastern College, striving for the establishment of pharmacological education, with the aim of differentiating medicine and pharmacology. In March 1872, the Meiji emperor's visit to the Eastern College took place, and as the new academic system was implemented on August 3, the Eastern College was renamed First University District Medical School. In November 1875, as his employment contract came to its term, Muller returned to his homeland. The photograph captures foreign instructors enjoying some entertainment. Muller stands on the right side.

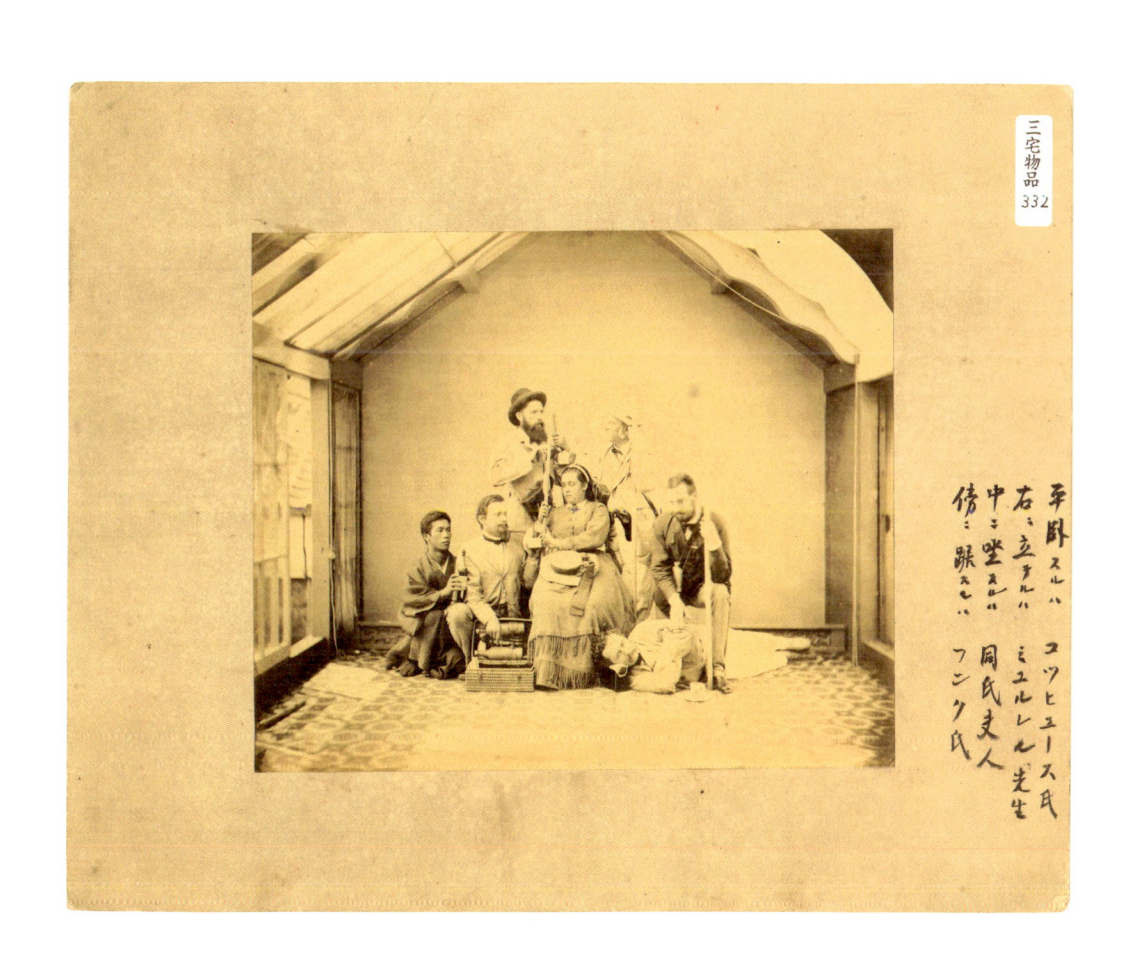

平臥スルハ　コツヒユース氏
右ニ立ツルハ　ミユルレル「先生」
中ニ坐スルハ　同氏夫人
傍ニ蹲スルハ　フンク氏

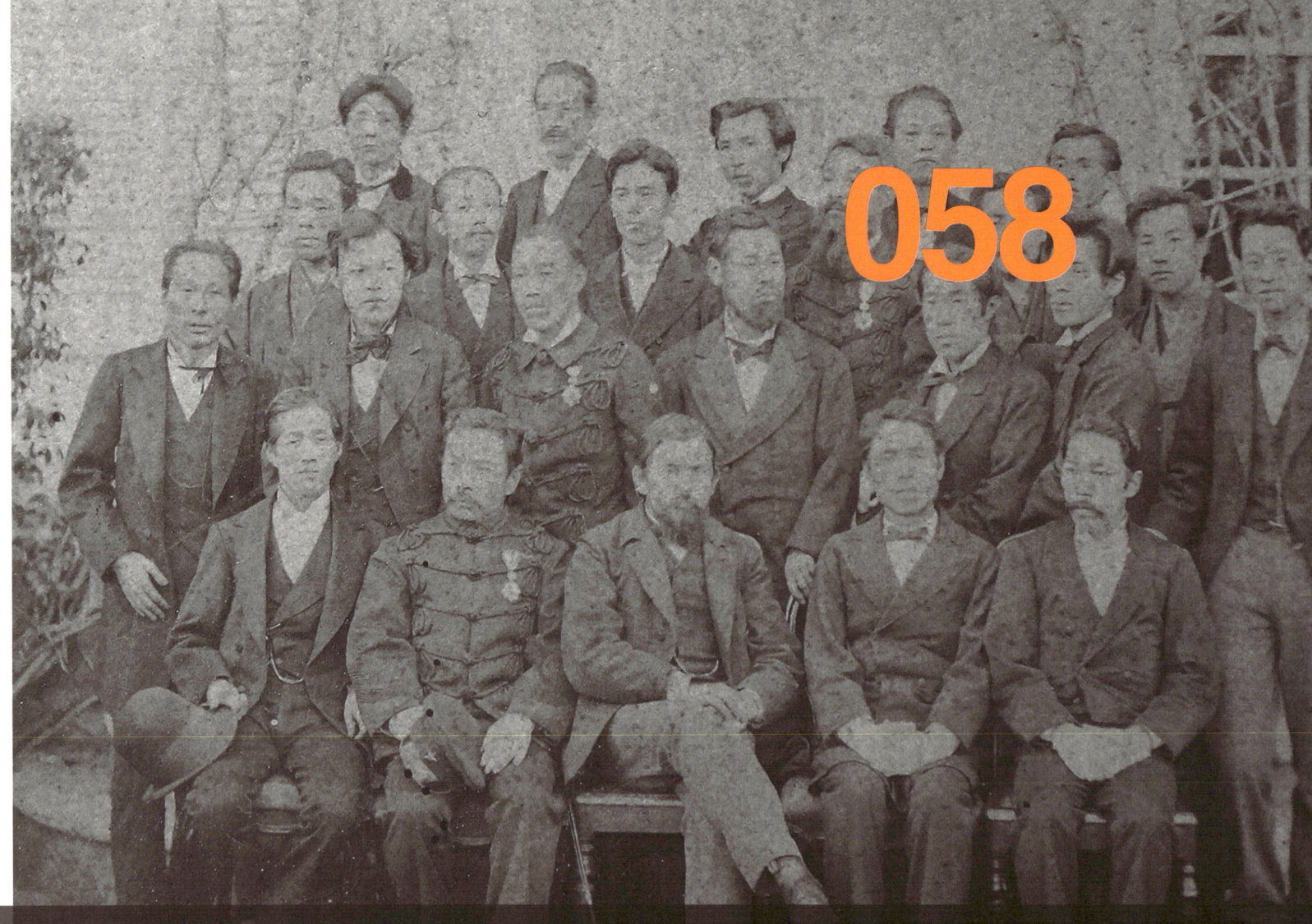

シュルツェ送別会写真

明治14(1881)年／松崎晋二撮影／鶏卵紙写真、厚紙台紙貼り／本紙縦205、横265、台紙縦355、横435、封紙縦520、横385／東京大学総合研究博物館所蔵三宅コレクション

台紙表に「東京湯島松崎晋二製麹町紀尾井町分店」の印字あり。封紙表に「此写真ハ『シエルツエ』教師帰国送別ノ際撮影セシモノニテ即チ教師ノ左二着席セラルハ桐原先生ナリ教師ノ右ニアリテ軍服ヲ着セラルハ池田先生ナリ」の墨書あり。エミル・シュルツェ(1840–1924)はベルリンの軍医学校に学び、普仏戦争に従軍したのち、キングス・カレッジ・ロンドンの臨床外科教授ジョゼフ・リスター(1827–1912)の許で石灰酸消毒法を学び、ドイツに「リスター法」を広めたことで知られる。明治7(1874)年12月、のちに東京大学初代医学部総理を拝命する池田謙齋(1841–1918)の依頼を受けて来日し、外科医として東京医学校の教育を率いている。明治14(1881)年に無事任期を満了し、帰国している。東京中橋和泉町の写真師松崎晋二(1850–没年未詳)の撮った写真は、送別会のときのものと思われる。帰国するシュルツェに西陣織が贈られたのは、このときのことであろう。

Photograph of Schultze's Farewell Reception

1881 / Taken by Shinji Matsuzaki / Photograph on albumen paper, mounted on cardboard / Photograph: L205, W265; Cardboard: L355, W435; Wrapping paper: L520, W385 / Miyake collection, UMUT

"Made by Shinji Matsuzaki, Yushima, Tokyo. Kojimachi Kioicho Annex" printed in Japanese on the back of the cardboard. "This photograph was taken upon instructor Schultze's farewell reception. Seated on his left is doctor Kirihara, and on his right in military uniform is doctor Ikeda" written in Japanese in ink on the recto of the wrapping paper. Emil August Wilhelm Schultze (1840 – 1924) studied at the Berlin Military School of Medicine, and after serving in the Franco-Prussian War, he studied the carbolic acid sterilization method under Joseph Lister (1827 – 1912), professor of Clinic Surgery at King's College, London. He is known for having generalized the Lister method in Germany. In December 1874, he came to Japan upon the demand of Kensei Ikeda (1841 – 1918), who was later to be named first director of the Faculty of Medicine of the University of Tokyo, and took in charge education at the Tokyo School of Medicine as a surgeon. In 1881, as his contract came to term, he returned to his homeland. This photograph, taken by Shinji Matsuzaki (1850 – date unknown) who had his studio in Nakahashi Izumicho, Tokyo, is thought to capture Schultze's farewell reception. It is probably at this time that a Nishijin silk fabric was offered to him.

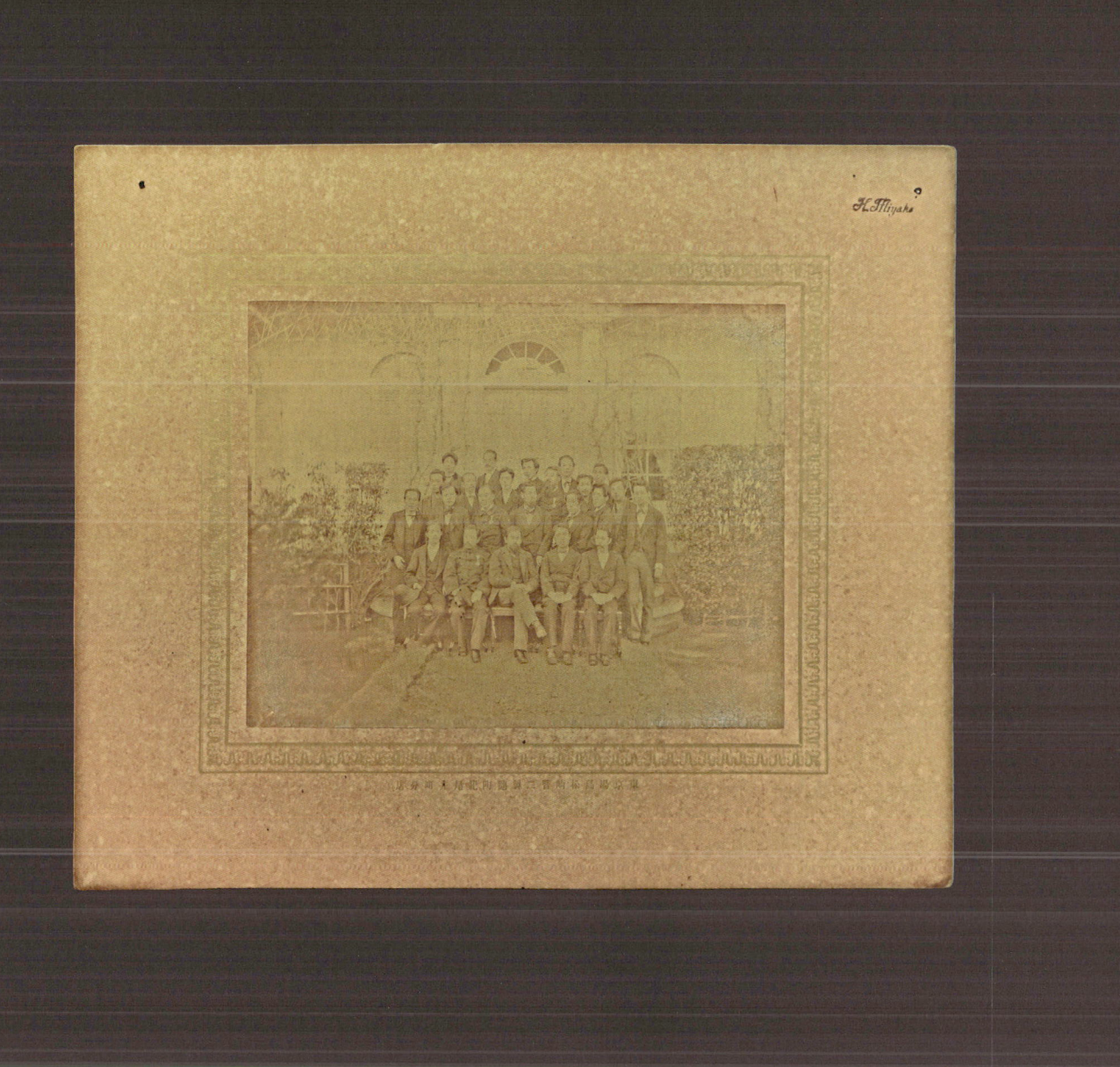

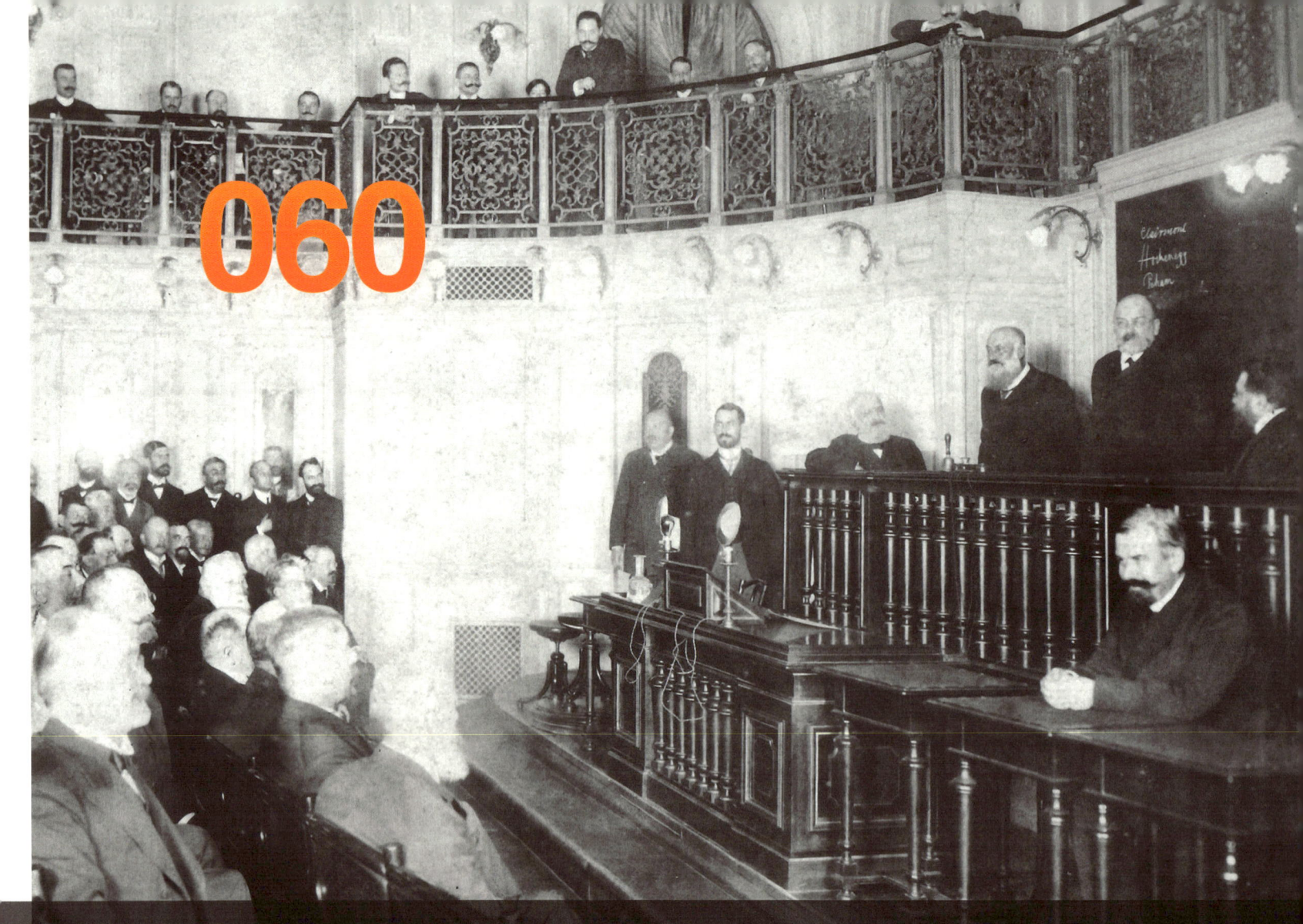

講演会写真
明治26(1893)年／チャールズ・スコリック撮影／鶏卵紙写真、厚紙台紙貼り／本紙縦206、横258、台紙縦247、横325／東京大学総合研究博物館所蔵三宅コレクション

台紙に貼付。詳細未詳。台紙表には「CHARLES SCOLIK k.u.k.Hof-Photograph」「WIEN VIII. Piaristengasse 48.」の印字があり、裏面には鉛筆で「fl. 1000 53.00 / 1893 erfaut」「Charles Scolik k.u.k.Hof-Photograph / Wien」とある。チャールズ・スコリック(1854－1928)はウィーンの写真家。

Photograph of a Conference
1893 / Taken by Charles Scolik / Photograph on albumen paper, mounted on cardboard / Photograph: L206, W258; Cardboard: L247, W325 / Miyake collection, UMUT

Details unknown. The cardboard bears on its recto the printed mention "Charles Scolik k.u.k.Hof-Photograph / Wien VIII. Piaristengasse 48." The mentions "fl. 1000 53.00 / 1893 erfaut" and "Charles Scolik k.u.k.Hof-Photograph / Wien" are written in pencil on the back. Charles Scolik (1854 – 1928) was a photographer established in Wien.

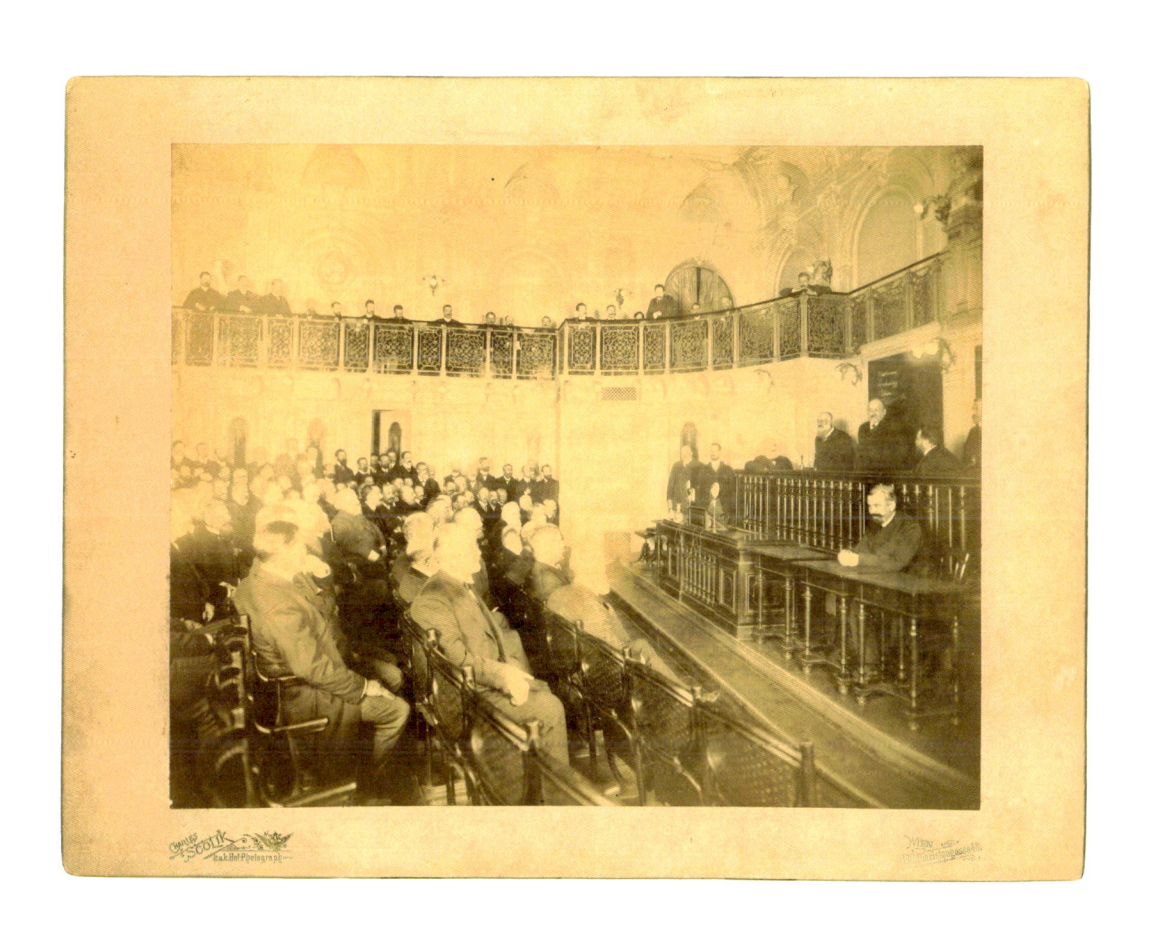

062

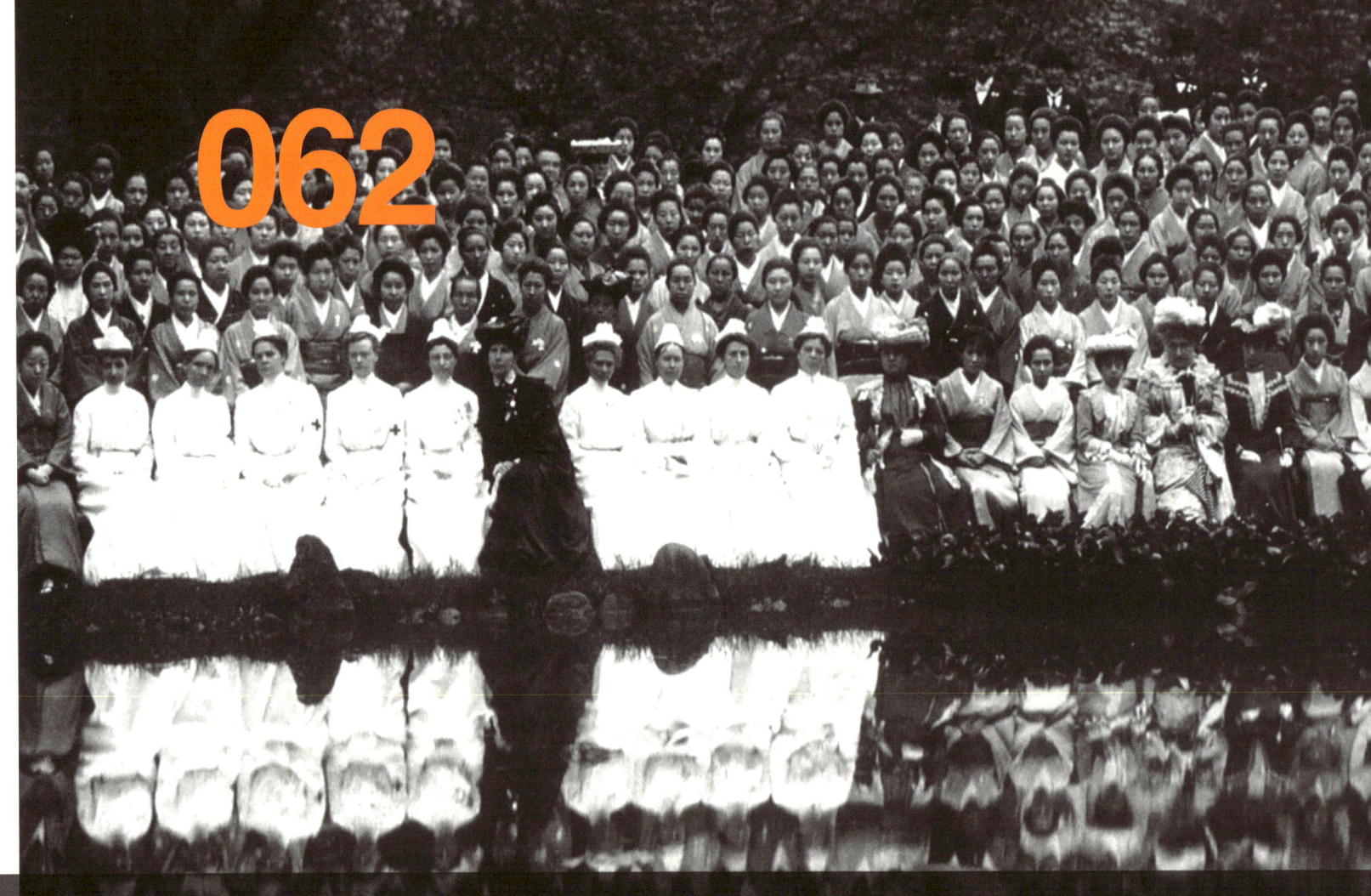

マッギー夫人歓迎会写真
明治37(1904)年／佐藤福待撮影／ゼラチンシルバープリント、厚紙台紙貼り／本紙縦269、横397、台紙縦421、横548／東京大学総合研究博物館所蔵三宅コレクション

台紙表印字「米国写真学士佐藤福待撮影」「TAKEN BY H.F.SATOW G.I.C.P.」、裏墨書「明治卅七年マッギー夫人歓迎会　後楽園ニ於テ撮影」。米西戦争看護婦会会長アニータ・ニューカム・マッギー(1864–1940)は日露戦争への万国赤十字社の医療支援活動の一環として明治37(1904)年に来日している。この歓迎会の様子は、映像記録でも残されている。

Photograph of Anita McGee's Welcome Reception
1904 / Taken by Fukuji Sato / Gelatin silver print, mounted on cardboard / Photograph: L269, W397; Cardboard: L421, W548 / Miyake collection, UMUT

"Taken by H.F.Satow G.I.C.P." printed in Japanese and English on the cardboard recto. On the back, "Welcome reception of McGee in the 37th year of Meiji, at Korakuen" written in Japanese in ink. Anita Newcomb McGee (1864 – 1940), president of the Society of Spanish-American War Nurses, visited Japan in 1904 in the context of the International Red Cross support to the Russo-Japanese War. Film footage of this welcome reception also remains.

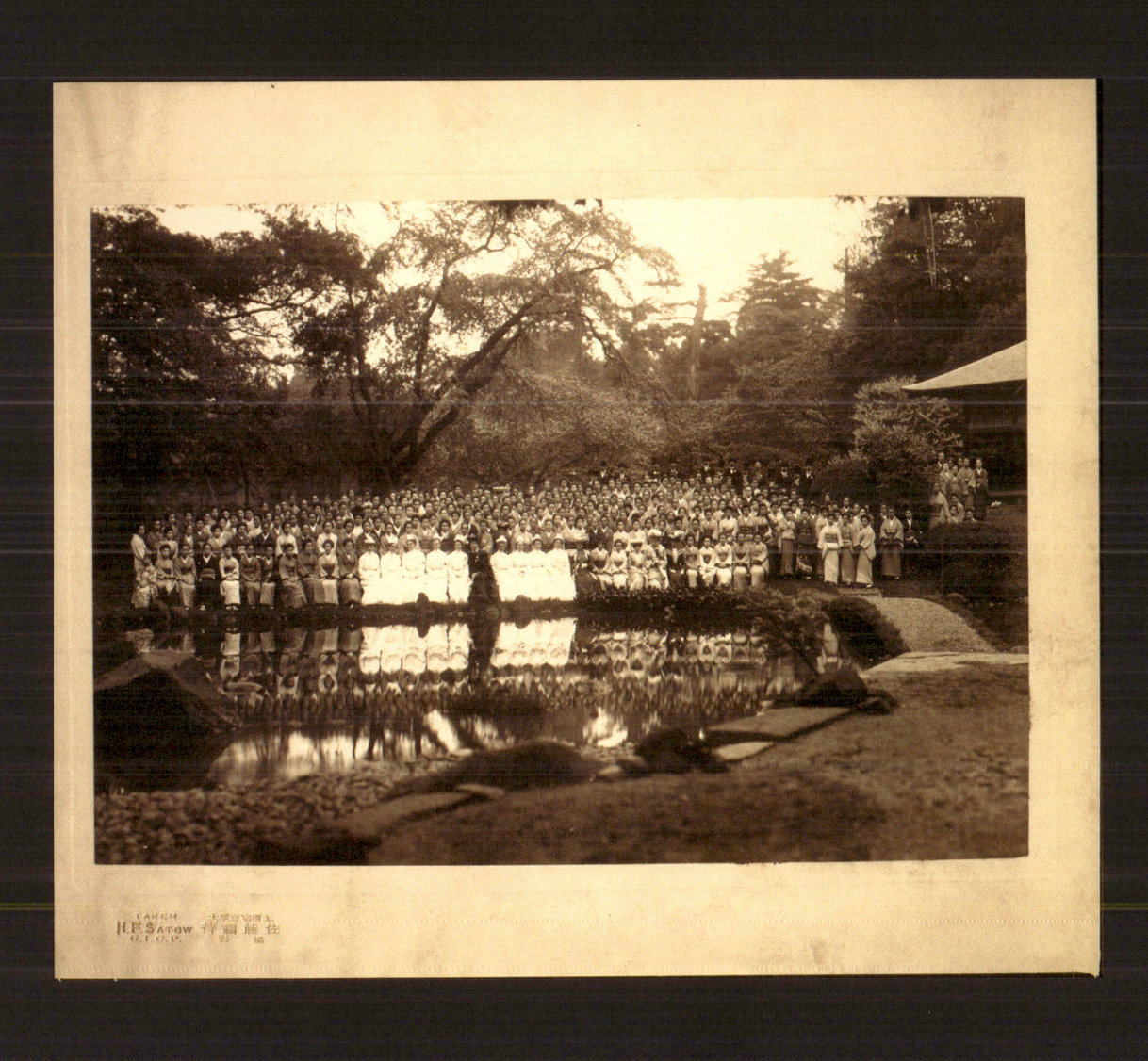

064

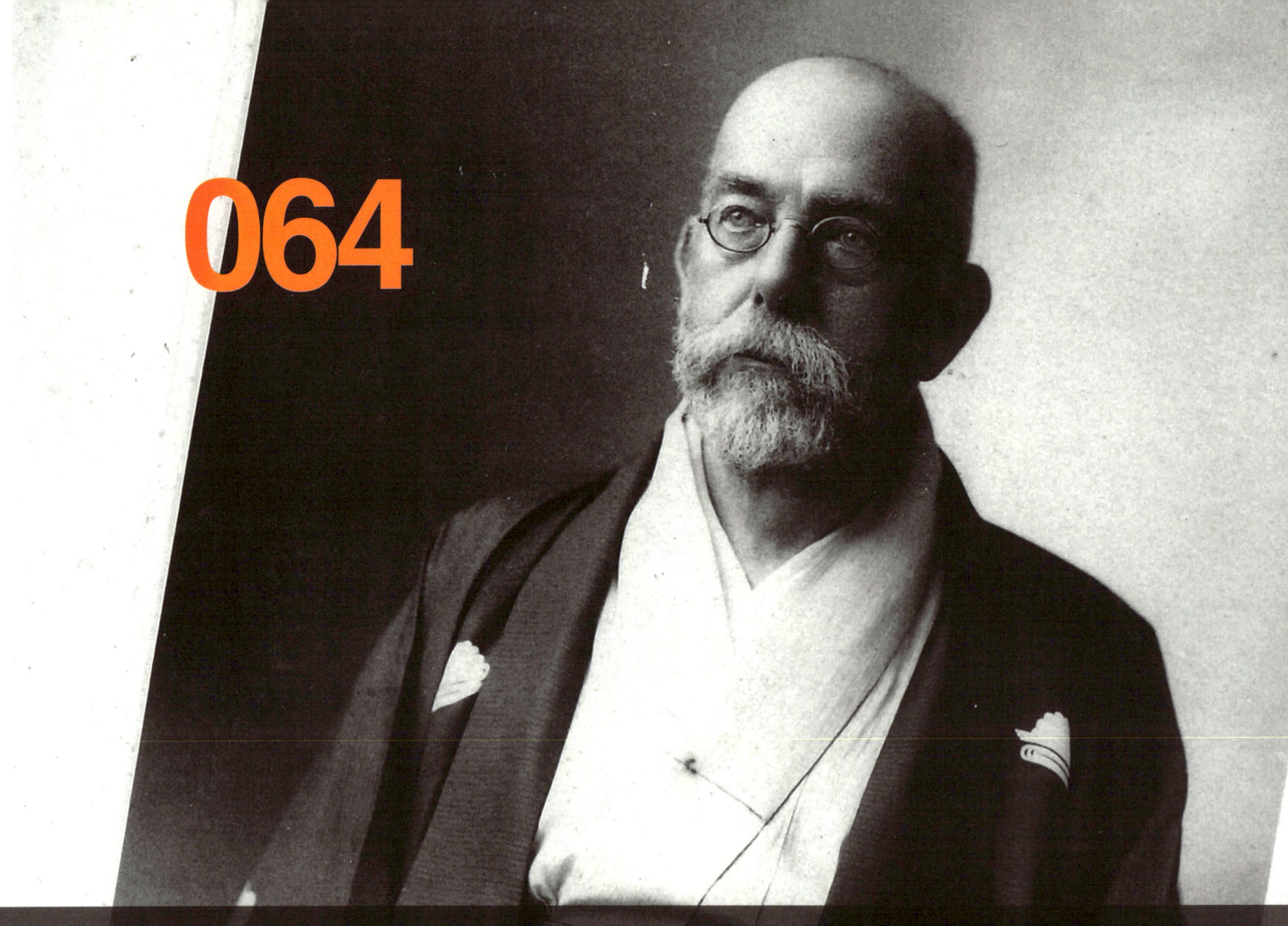

コッホ写真
明治41（1908）年／小川一眞印行／紙焼き写真／縦273、横205／東京大学総合研究博物館所蔵 三宅コレクション

ロベルト・コッホ（1843-1910）は、炭疽菌、結核菌、コレラ菌を発見した細菌学者で、1905年、結核に関する研究でノーベル生理学・医学賞を受賞している。破傷風菌の純粋培養に成功し、ペスト菌を発見した北里柴三郎（1853-1931）は、明治19（1886）年1月、ベルリン大学のコッホ研究室に入り、研究活動を始めている。明治32（1899）年4月、内務省の管轄となった国立伝染病研究所（東大医科学研究所の前身）の所長に就任し、明治41（1908）年6月、恩師のコッホ夫妻の訪日を実現している。写真は、のちに帝室技芸員となる写真家小川一眞（1860-1929）が撮影したものである。

Photograph of Koch
1908 / Published by Kazuma Ogawa / Photograph on printing paper / L273, W205 / Miyake collection, UMUT

Heinrich Hermann Robert Koch (1834 – 1910), a bacteriologist who discovered the *Bacillus anthracis*, the *Mycobacterium tuberculosis* and the *Vibrio cholerae*, was the recipient of the 1905 Nobel Prize in Physiology or Medicine for his research on tuberculosis. Shibasaburo Kitazato (1853 – 1931), who succeeded in growing the tetanus bacillus in pure culture and discovered the *Yersinia pestis*, started his research at Koch's laboratory at the University of Berlin in January 1886. In April 1899, Kitazato was appointed director of the National Institute of Infectious Diseases (which was later to become the Institute of Medical Science of the University of Tokyo), which was then under control of the Home Ministry, and succeeded in organizing the Koch couple's visit to Japan in June 1908. The photograph was taken by Kazuma Ogawa (1860 – 1929), who was later to be named court artist.

R. Koch.

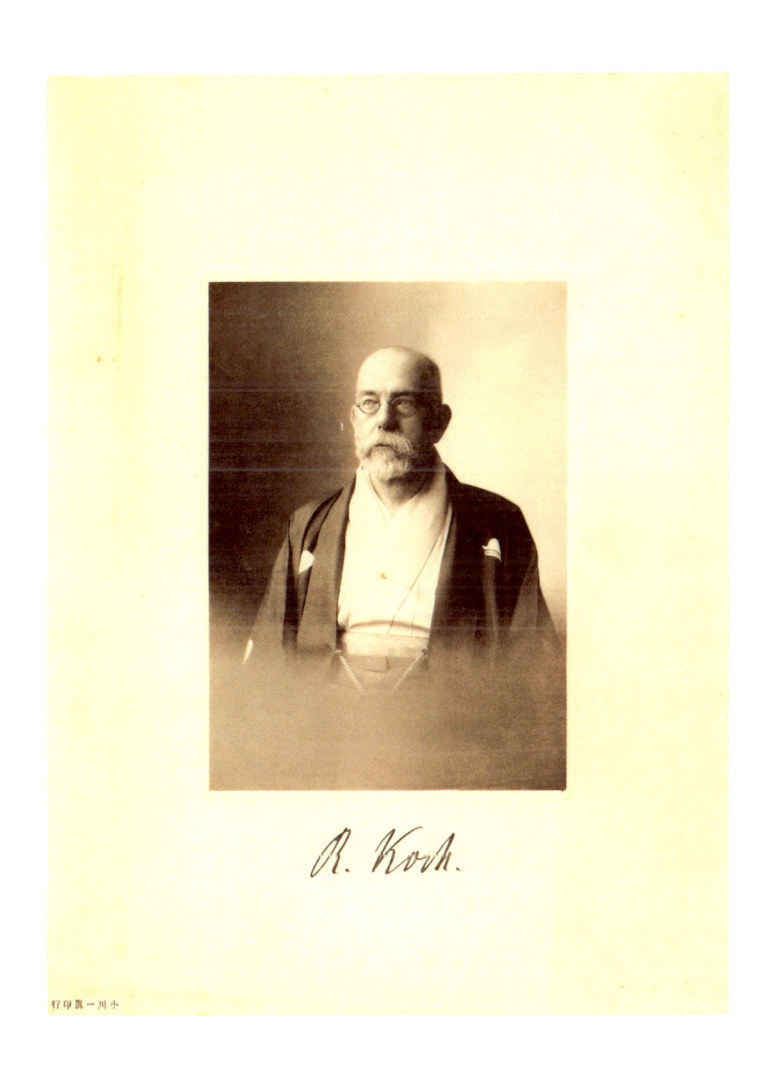

Collection of Educational Wall Charts

Wall charts have been used as an educational tool since the beginning of the Meiji period. They were hung on the wall surrounding the platform, and teachers gave explanations by pointing to each part of the wall chart. Wall charts were thus an indispensable educational tool. Some wall charts are mounted on a scroll, while others are printed on cardboard. Many images used for wall charts were reproduced from European monographs and illustrated reference books. Universities fully employed illustrators who were specialized in such work. Along with professional illustrators, some students from the Tokyo Art School also took part in this work to earn some pocket money, and some of the extrant wall charts present a high artistic value. Sadly, wall charts, which are now nothing more than a white elephant in educational institutions, have been mostly discarded.

教育用掛図コレクション

　掛図はヴィジュアル教育ツールとして、明治の初めから教育の現場で使われてきた。教壇の壁にこれを掛け、教師が指し棒で指示しながら解説を施す。昔日の教育風景になくてはならない教育ツールであった。実際に壁に掛けて使われたことから「掛図」と呼び慣わされるようになった。掛図には軸装のものと厚紙のものがある。掛図に描出された絵柄の多くは、ヨーロッパの研究書や図譜から転写されたものである。大学はその種の作業を専門とする画工を専属として抱えていた。専属画工たちに混じって東京美術学校の学生たちも、小遣い稼ぎに掛図制作を請け負っていたようで、残されている掛図のなかには美術的創作物として質の高いものも散見される。ともあれ、今日の教育現場では無用の長物と化した掛図は、多くが廃棄処分の憂き目にあっている。

068

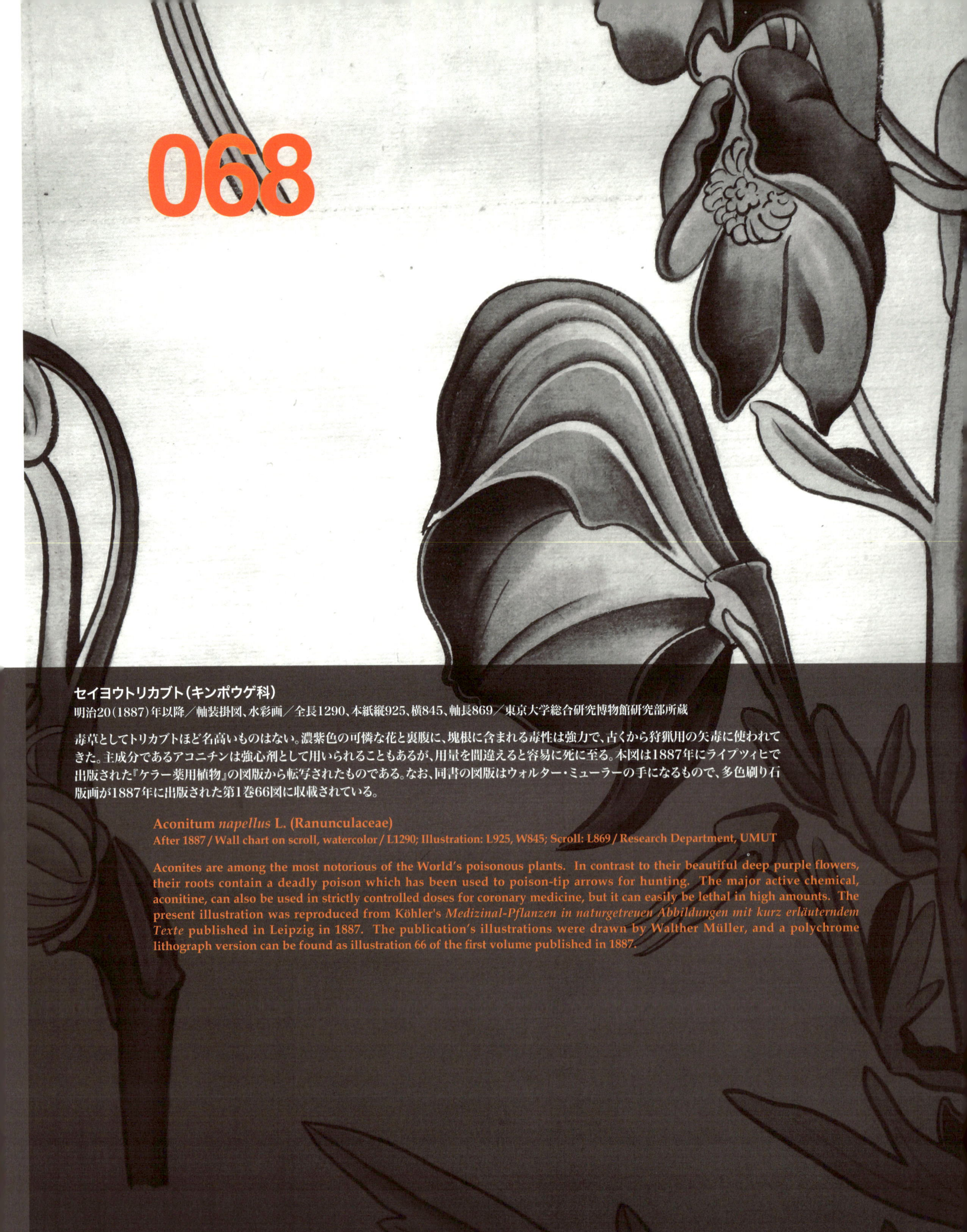

セイヨウトリカブト（キンポウゲ科）
明治20(1887)年以降／軸装掛図、水彩画／全長1290、本紙縦925、横845、軸長869／東京大学総合研究博物館研究部所蔵

毒草としてトリカブトほど名高いものはない。濃紫色の可憐な花と裏腹に、塊根に含まれる毒性は強力で、古くから狩猟用の矢毒に使われてきた。主成分であるアコニチンは強心剤として用いられることもあるが、用量を間違えると容易に死に至る。本図は1887年にライプツィヒで出版された『ケラー薬用植物』の図版から転写されたものである。なお、同書の図版はウォルター・ミューラーの手になるもので、多色刷り石版画が1887年に出版された第1巻66図に収載されている。

Aconitum *napellus* L. (Ranunculaceae)
After 1887 / Wall chart on scroll, watercolor / L1290; Illustration: L925, W845; Scroll: L869 / Research Department, UMUT

Aconites are among the most notorious of the World's poisonous plants. In contrast to their beautiful deep purple flowers, their roots contain a deadly poison which has been used to poison-tip arrows for hunting. The major active chemical, aconitine, can also be used in strictly controlled doses for coronary medicine, but it can easily be lethal in high amounts. The present illustration was reproduced from Köhler's *Medizinal-Pflanzen in naturgetreuen Abbildungen mit kurz erläuterndem Texte* published in Leipzig in 1887. The publication's illustrations were drawn by Walther Müller, and a polychrome lithograph version can be found as illustration 66 of the first volume published in 1887.

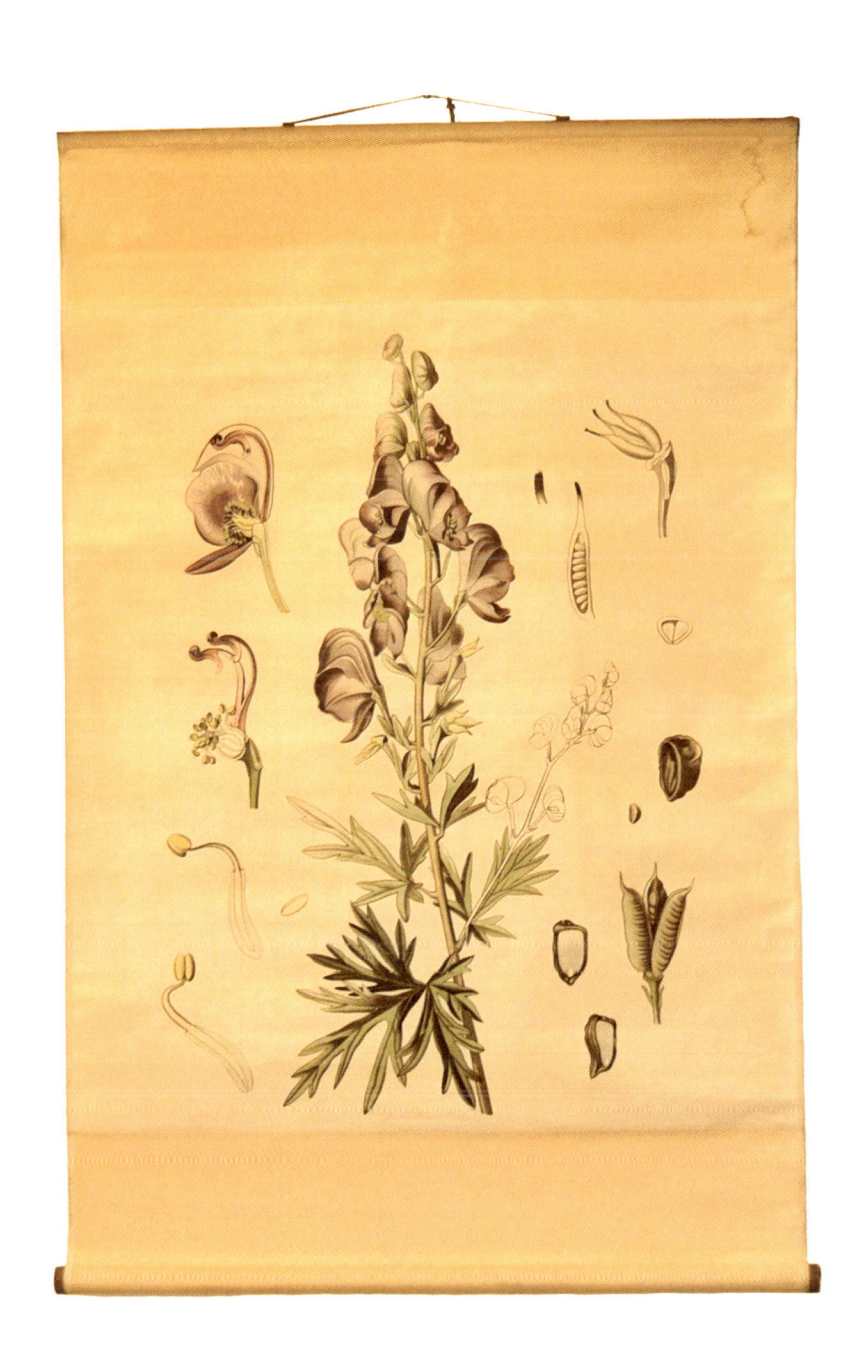

070

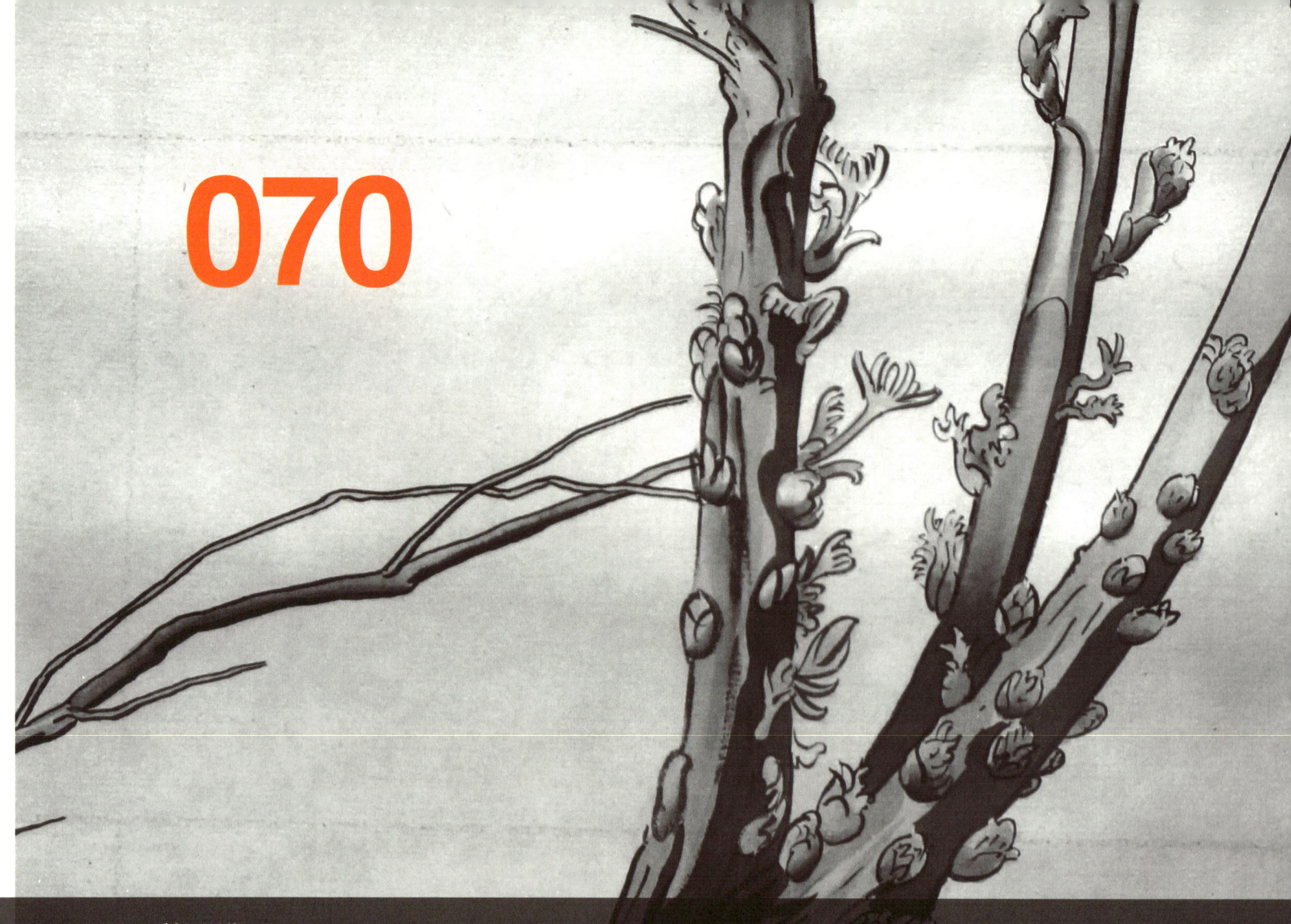

シナヨモギ（キク科）
明治23（1890）年以降／軸装掛図、水彩画／全長1255、本紙縦840、横855、軸長870／東京大学総合研究博物館研究部所蔵

ヨモギ類には有用なものが多い。草餅、アブサン酒、お灸のもぐさなど、その用途も多様である。シナヨモギは中央アジアに分布する。蕾には回虫駆除に効果のあるサントニンが多く含まれる。日本でも、かつてはサントニン精製を目的として、本種や近縁なミブヨモギが盛んに栽培されていた。本図は1887年にライプツィヒで出版された『ケラー薬用植物』の図版から転写されたものである。なお、同書の図版はウォルター・ミューラーの手になるもので、多色刷り石版画が1890年以降に出版された第2巻196図に収載されている。

Seriphidium cinum (Bergius ex Poljak.) Poljak. (Compositae)
After 1890 / Wall chart on scroll, watercolor / L1255; Illustration: L840, W855; Scroll: L870 / Research Department, UMUT

Artemisia is a genus containing many useful plants. For example, leaves of several species are used to make herb rice cakes, absinth, and moxa. The buds of *Seriphidium cinum*, which was formally recognized as a member of *Artemisia*, are rich in santonin and have been used to kill intestinal worms. *Seriphidium* was once widely cultivated in Japan, especially when night soil was used as fertilizer. The present illustration was reproduced from Köhler's *Medizinal-Pflanzen in naturgetreuen Abbildungen mit kurz erläuterndem Texte* published in Leipzig in 1887. The publication's illustrations were drawn by Walther Müller, and a polychrome lithograph version can be found as illustration 196 of the second volume published after 1890.

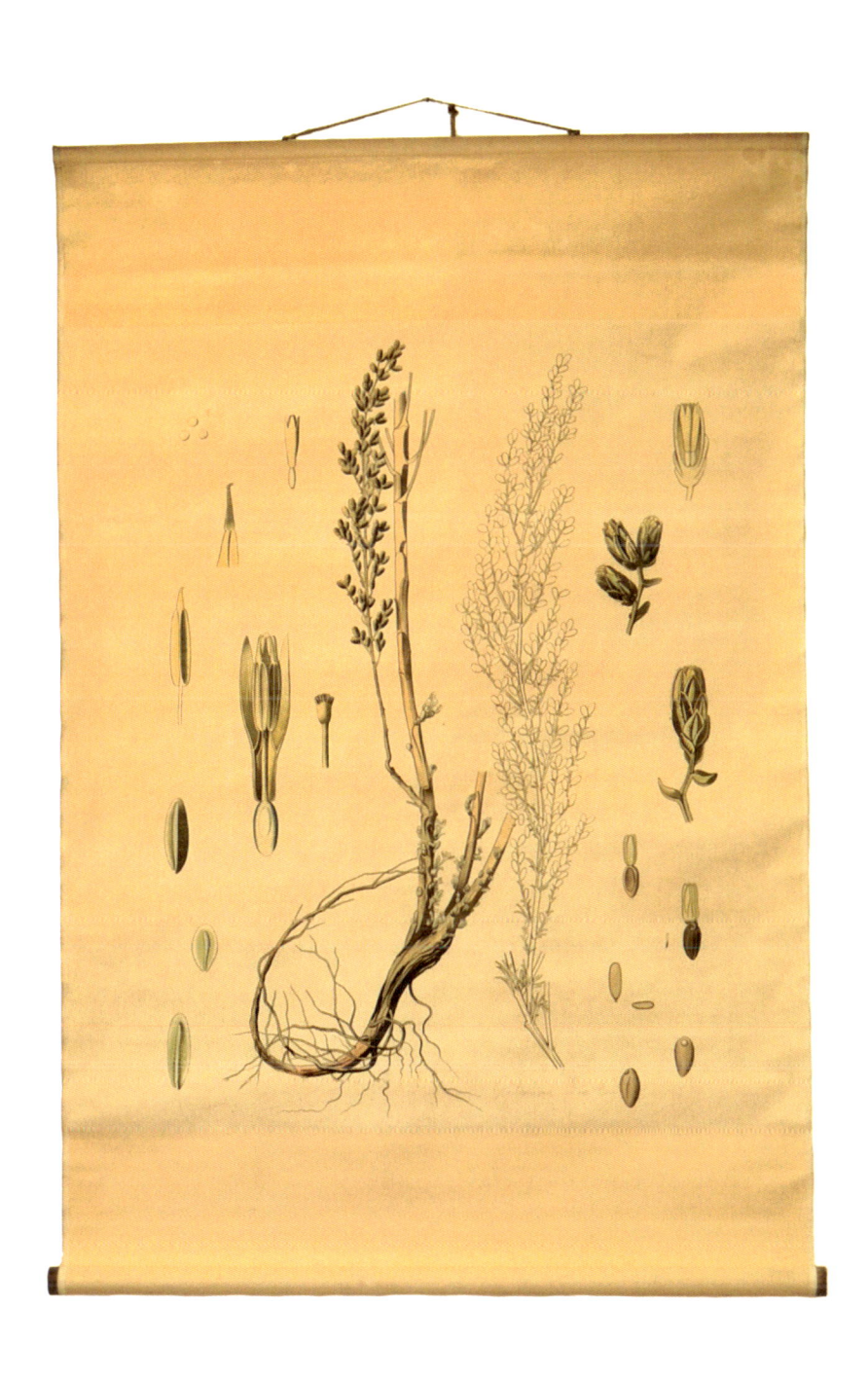

072

シロバナチョウセンアサガオ（ナス科）
明治23（1890）年以降／軸装掛図、水彩画／全長1270、本紙縦905、横840、軸長865／東京大学総合研究博物館研究部所蔵

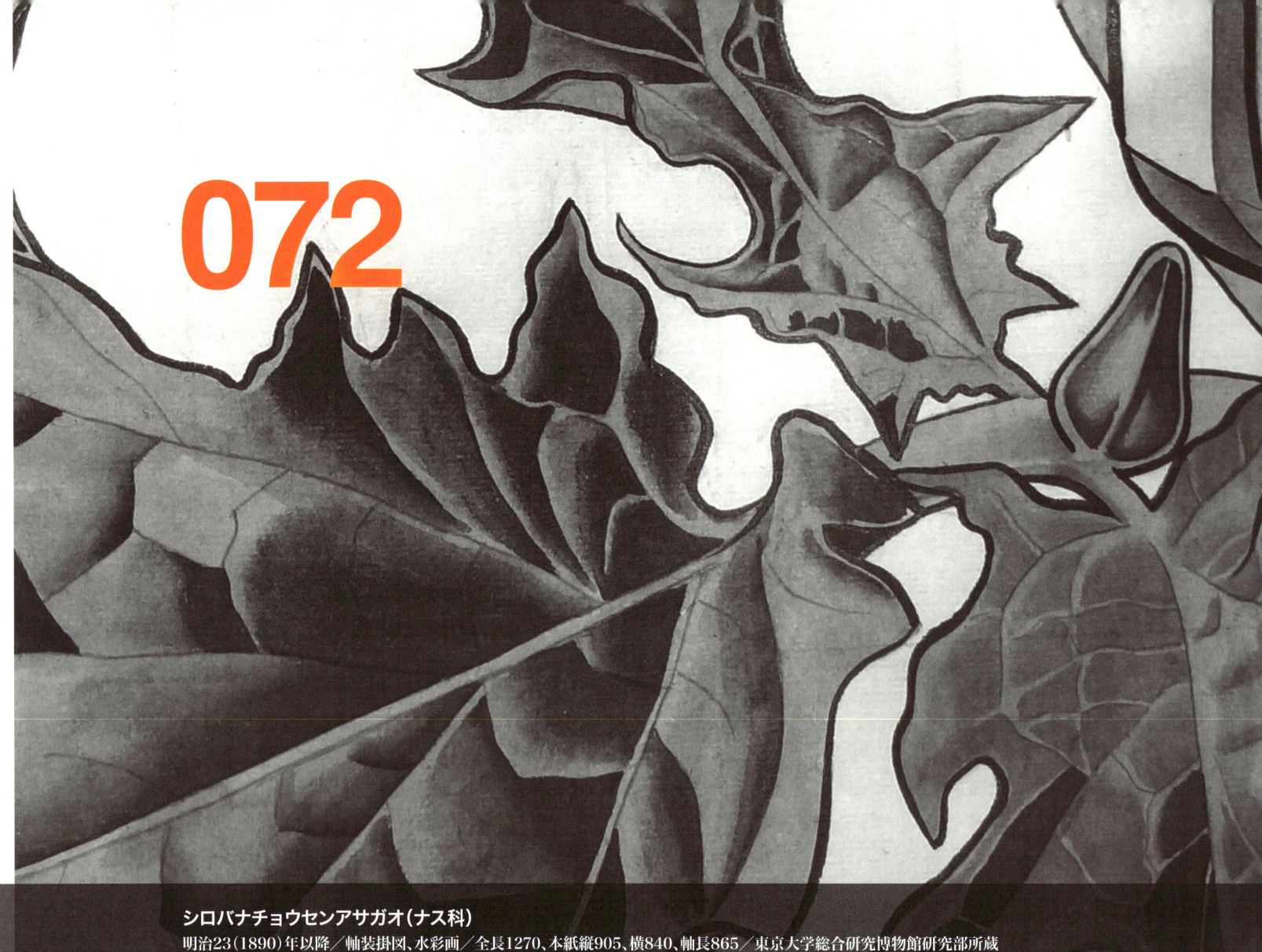

欧米で薬用に栽培されていた本種は、明治初め日本に将来され、現在では野生化している。夏から秋にかけ、トランペット状の大輪を咲かす。植物体全体にアルカロイド類を有する。種子に多く含まれるスコポラミンは、目薬や麻酔剤の原料として利用されている。本図は1887年にライプツィヒで出版された『ケラー薬用植物』の図版から転写されたものである。なお、同書の図版はウォルター・ミューラーの手になるもので、多色刷り石版画が1890年以降に出版された第2巻169図に収載されている。

Datura stramonium L. f. *stramonium* (Solanaceae)
After 1890 / Wall chart on scroll, watercolor / L1270; Illustration: L905, W840; Scroll: L865 / Research Department, UMUT

Datura stramonium has long been grown in Europe as a medicinal plant, and was imported to Japan during the Meiji period, where local groups of plants grew from stray seed. The big trumpet-like flowers open from summer to autumn in Japan. All parts of the plant contain alkaloids, especially the seeds which are rich in scopolamine. Scopolamine has been used for eye drops and as an anesthetic. The present illustration was reproduced from Köhler's *Medizinal-Pflanzen in naturgetreuen Abbildungen mit kurz erläuterndem Texte* published in Leipzig in 1887. The publication's illustrations were drawn by Walther Müller, and a polychrome lithograph version can be found as illustration 169 of the second volume published after 1890.

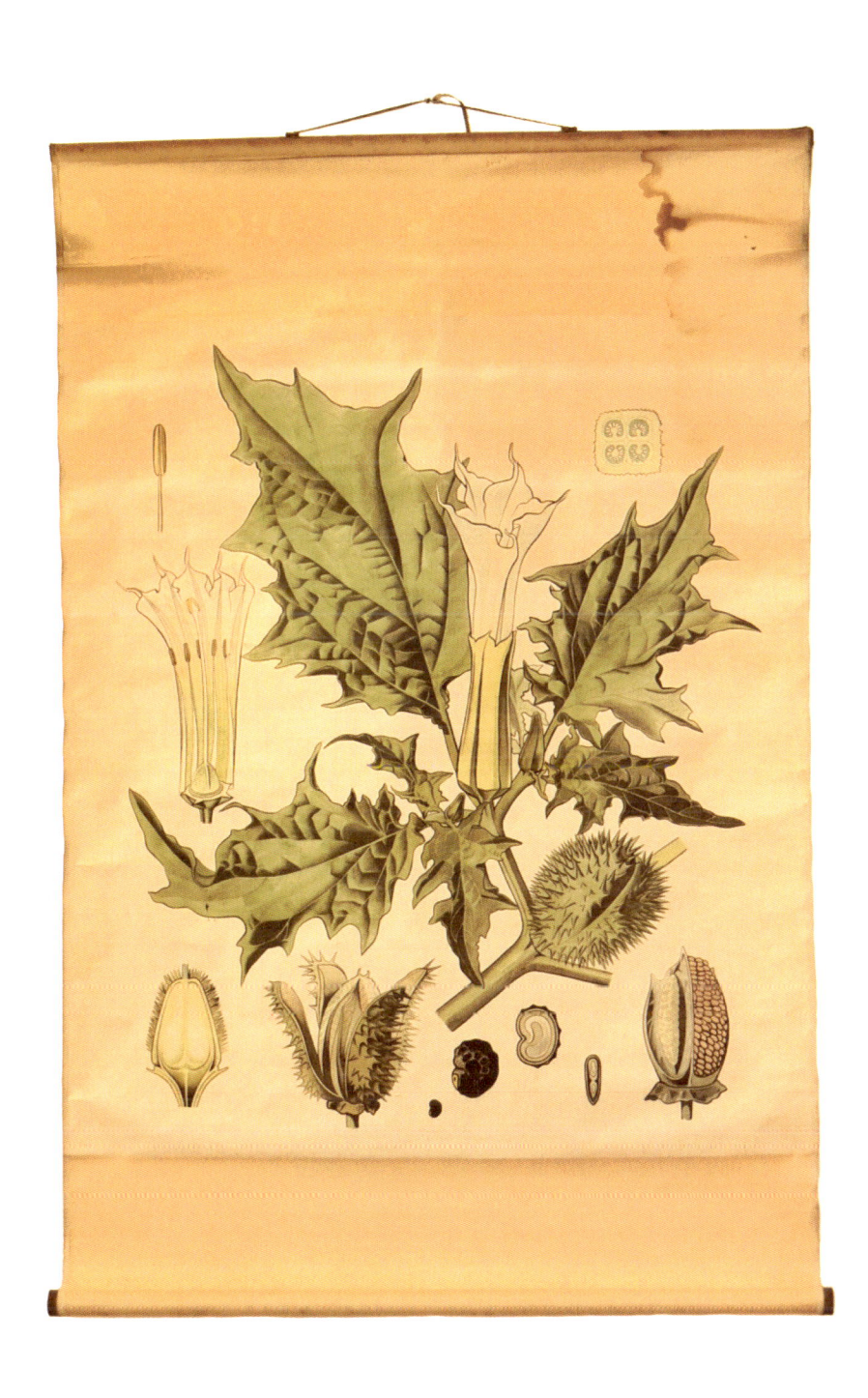

074

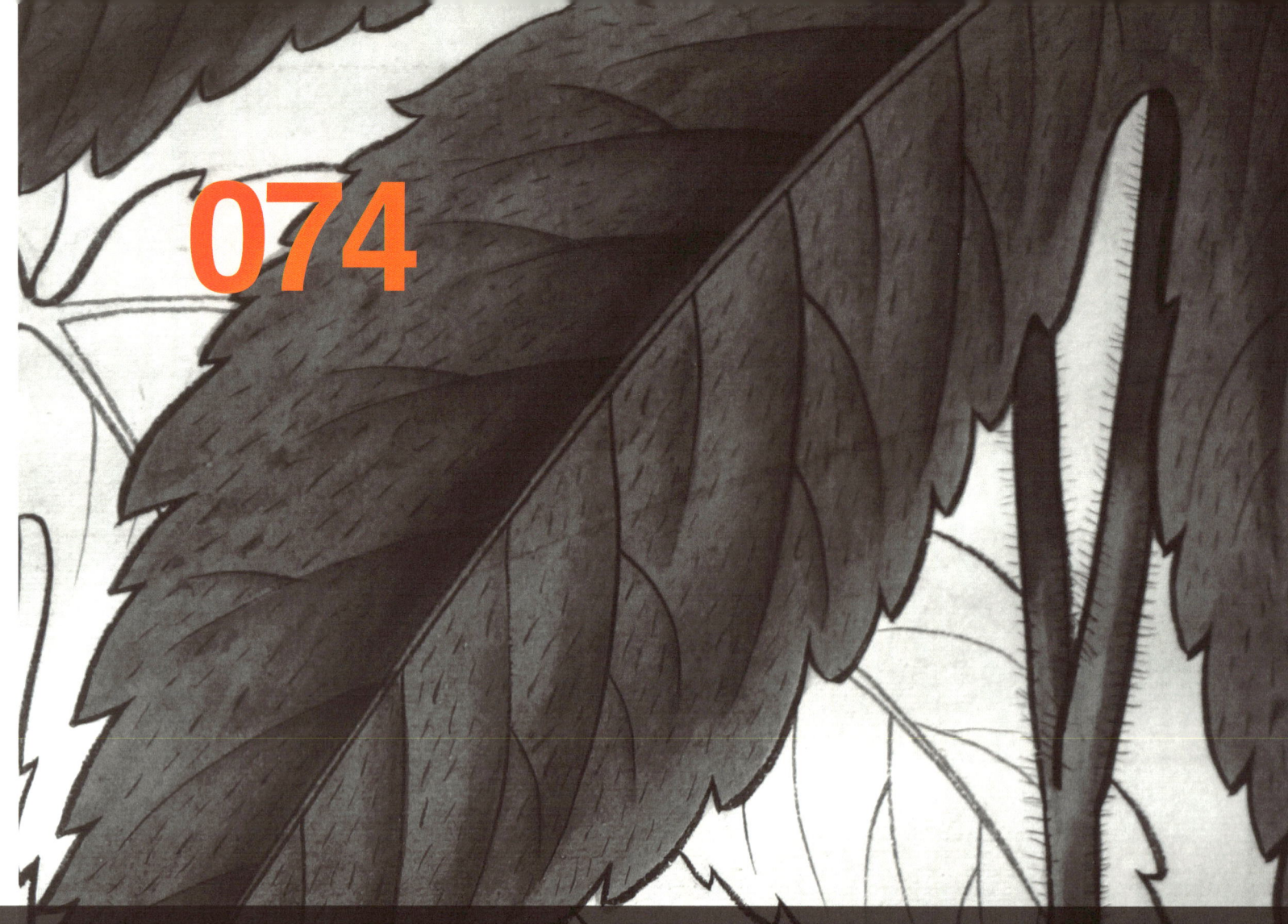

ゴールデンシール（キンポウゲ科）
明治20（1887）年以降／軸装掛図、水彩画／全長1310、本紙縦940、横843、軸長870／東京大学総合研究博物館研究部所蔵

北米原産の1属1種の多年生草本植物である。萼片は3枚で花弁は無く、雄しべと雌しべが多数ある。冬のあいだ地上部は枯れ、地下部のみが休眠状態になり、越冬する。根茎はヒドラスチス根とも呼ばれ、抗菌作用のある成分を多く含むことから、感染症予防に用いられる。本図は1887年にライプツィヒで出版された『ケラー薬用植物』の図版から転写されたものである。なお、同書の図版はウォルター・ミューラーの手になるもので、多色刷り石版画が1887年に出版された第1巻65図に収載されている。

Hydrastis Canadensis L. (Ranunculaceae)
After 1887 / Wall chart on scroll, watercolor / L1310; Illustration: L940, W843; Scroll: L870 / Research Department, UMUT

Hydrastis canadensis, a genus with just one species, is a perennial herb native to North America. The flower consists of three calyx lobes and many pistils and stamens, but no petals. In winter, the aerial parts of the plant die down and the underground parts, rhizome and root, survive in a dormant state. The rhizome - the "hydrastis root" – is used to guard against infectious diseases due to its antibacterial activity. The present illustration was reproduced from Köhler's *Medizinal-Pflanzen in naturgetreuen Abbildungen mit kurz erläuterndem Texte* published in Leipzig in 1887. The publication's illustrations were drawn by Walther Müller, and a polychrome lithograph version can be found as illustration 65 of the first volume published in 1887.

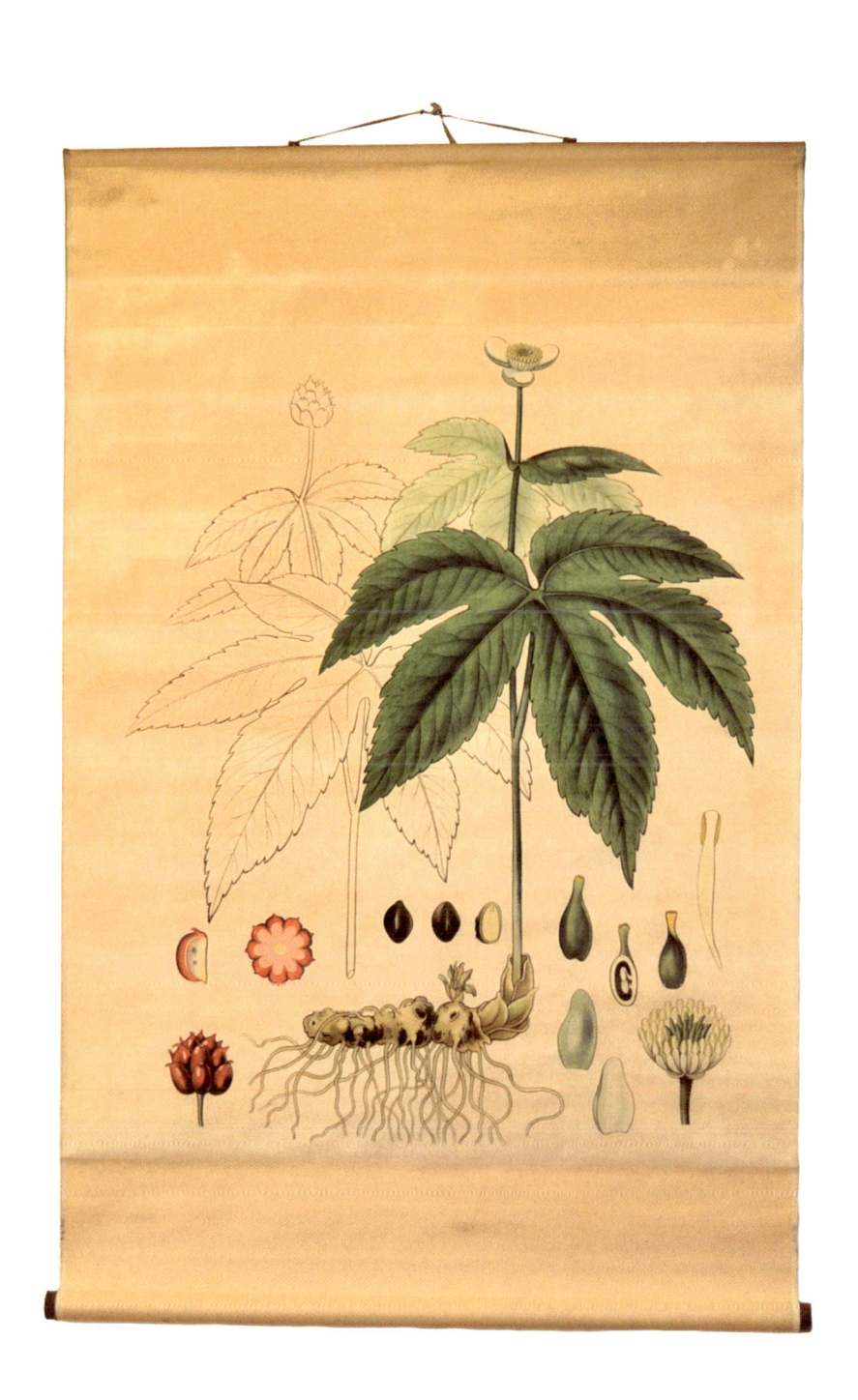

076

ベニテングタケ
明治20(1887)年以降／軸装掛図、水彩画／全長1300、本紙縦905、横826、軸長850／東京大学総合研究博物館研究部所蔵

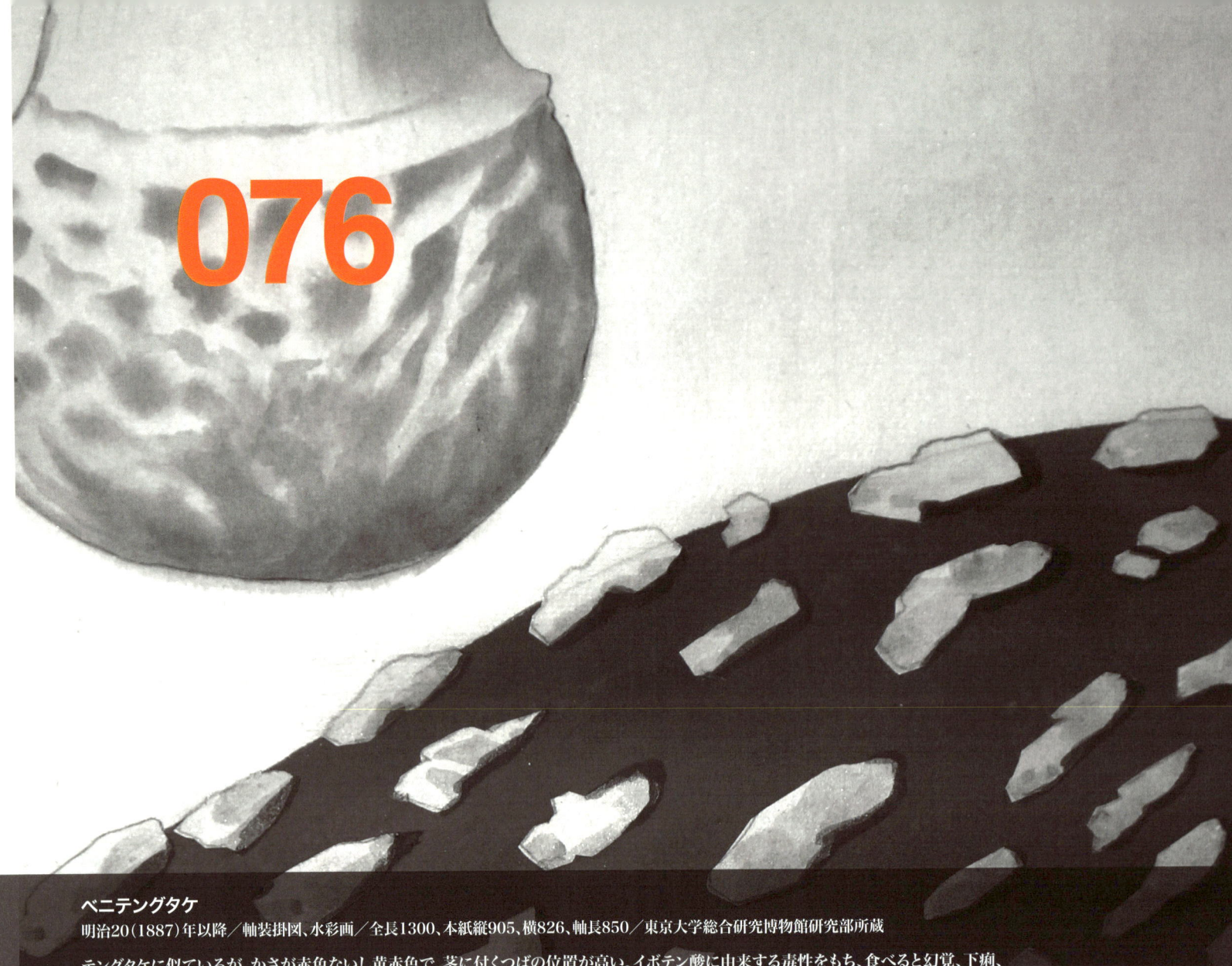

テングタケに似ているが、かさが赤色ないし黄赤色で、茎に付くつばの位置が高い。イボテン酸に由来する毒性をもち、食べると幻覚、下痢、嘔吐の症状を惹起する。ヨーロッパでは幸福の象徴とされ、クリスマスや新年の飾りのモチーフとなる。

Amanita muscarina (L.: Fr.) Lam.
After 1887 / Wall chart on scroll, watercolor / L1300; Illustration: L905, W826; Scroll: L850 / Research Department, UMUT

Amanita muscarina differs in the color of the pileus and the location of annulus from *A. pantherina*. These fungi contain the toxin ibotenic acid, which produces symptoms of hallucination, diarrhea and vomiting. Despite its toxicity, *A. muscarina* is considered as a symbol for happiness and used as a motif for Christmas and New Year celebrations.

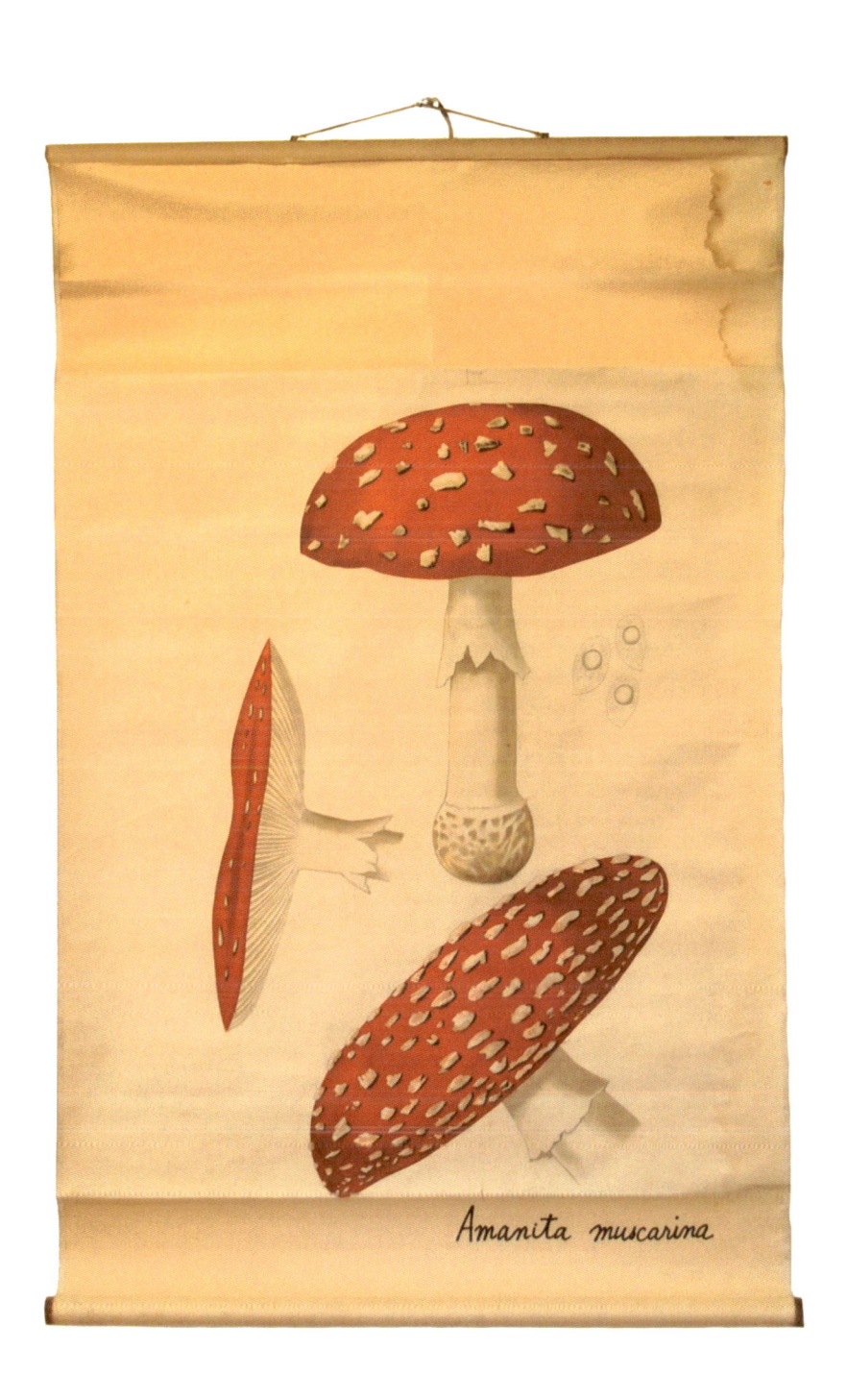

Amanita muscarina

078

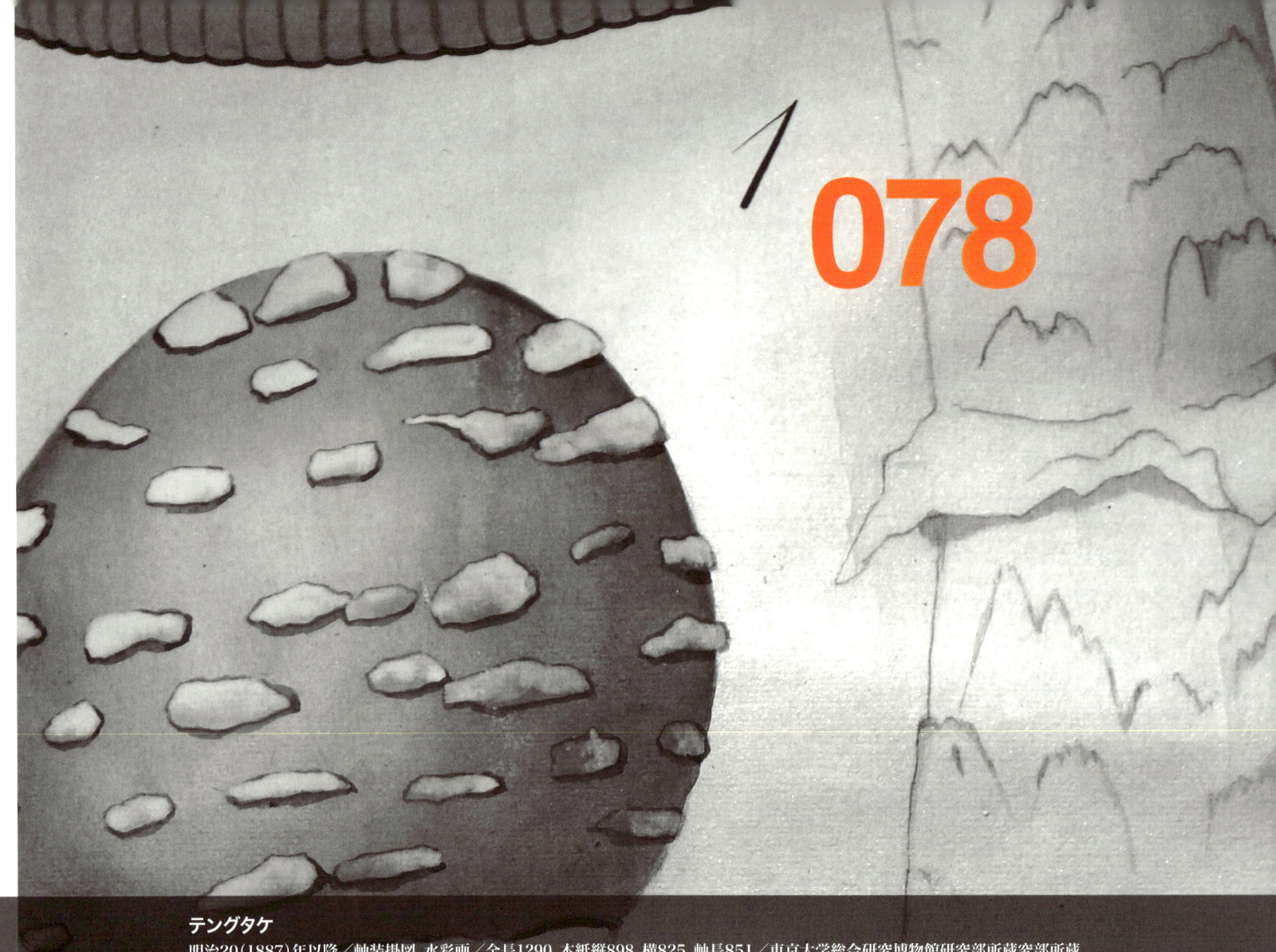

テングタケ
明治20(1887)年以降／軸装掛図、水彩画／全長1290、本紙縦898、横825、軸長851／東京大学総合研究博物館研究部所蔵

テングタケ科テングダケ属は国内で約40種が知られ、毒性をもつキノコを多く含む。本種は、かさの部分に、グルタミン酸と類似した化学構造をもつイボテン酸が多く含まれる。ハエが匂いに誘引され、そのかさを舐めたハエは動けなくなる。そのことからハエ取りに利用されてきた。

Amanita pantherina (L. : Fr.) Krombh.
After 1887 / Wall chart on scroll, watercolor / L1290; Illustration: L898, W825; Scroll: L851 / Research Department, UMUT

There are about 40 species in the genus *Amanita* (Amanitaceae) in Japan, and most contain chemical compounds that affect the activity of animals and may cause death. The pileus of *A. pantherina* contains ibotenic acid, which has a similar chemical constitution to glutamic acid. Drosophila flies are attracted by the aroma, but they are susceptible to ibotenic acid.

Amanita pantherina

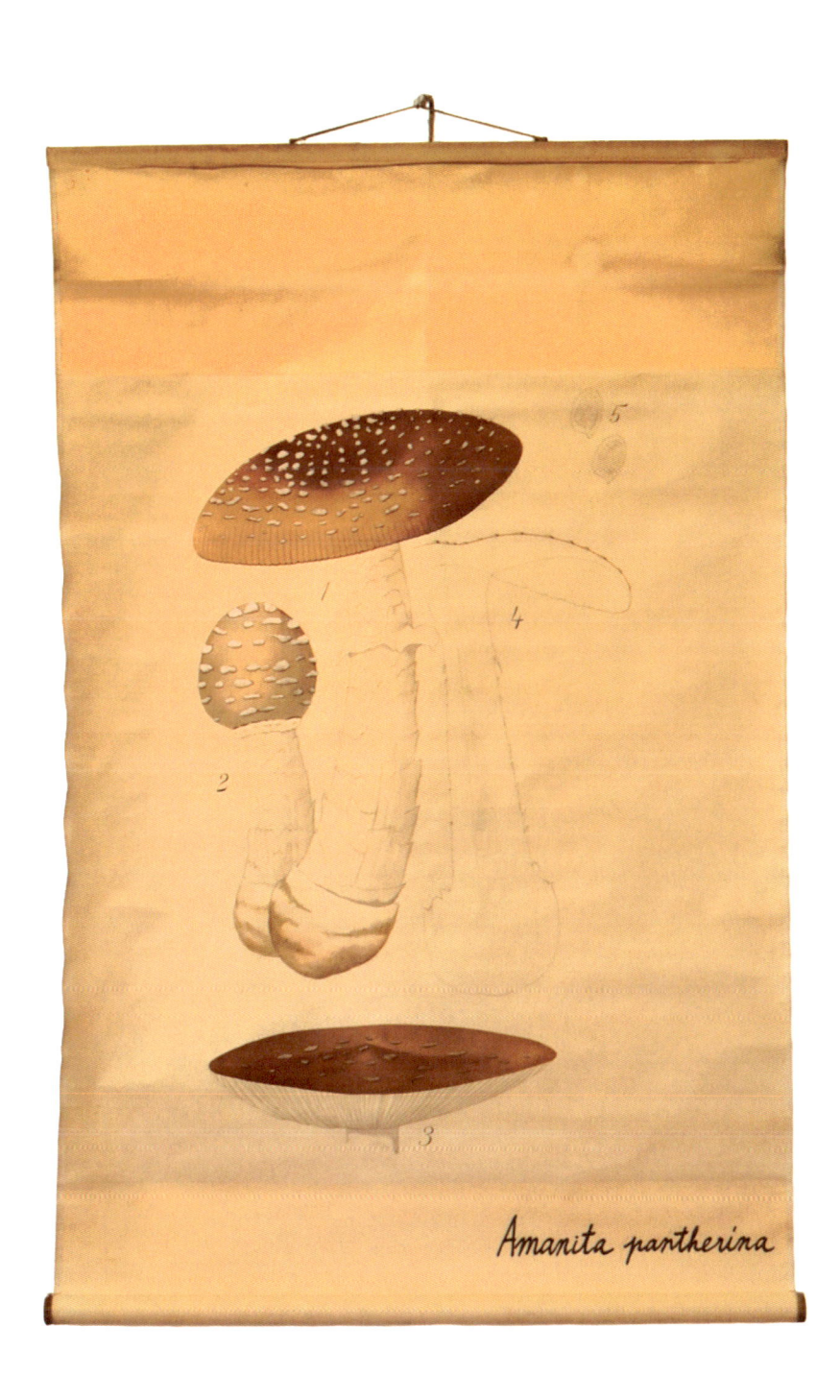

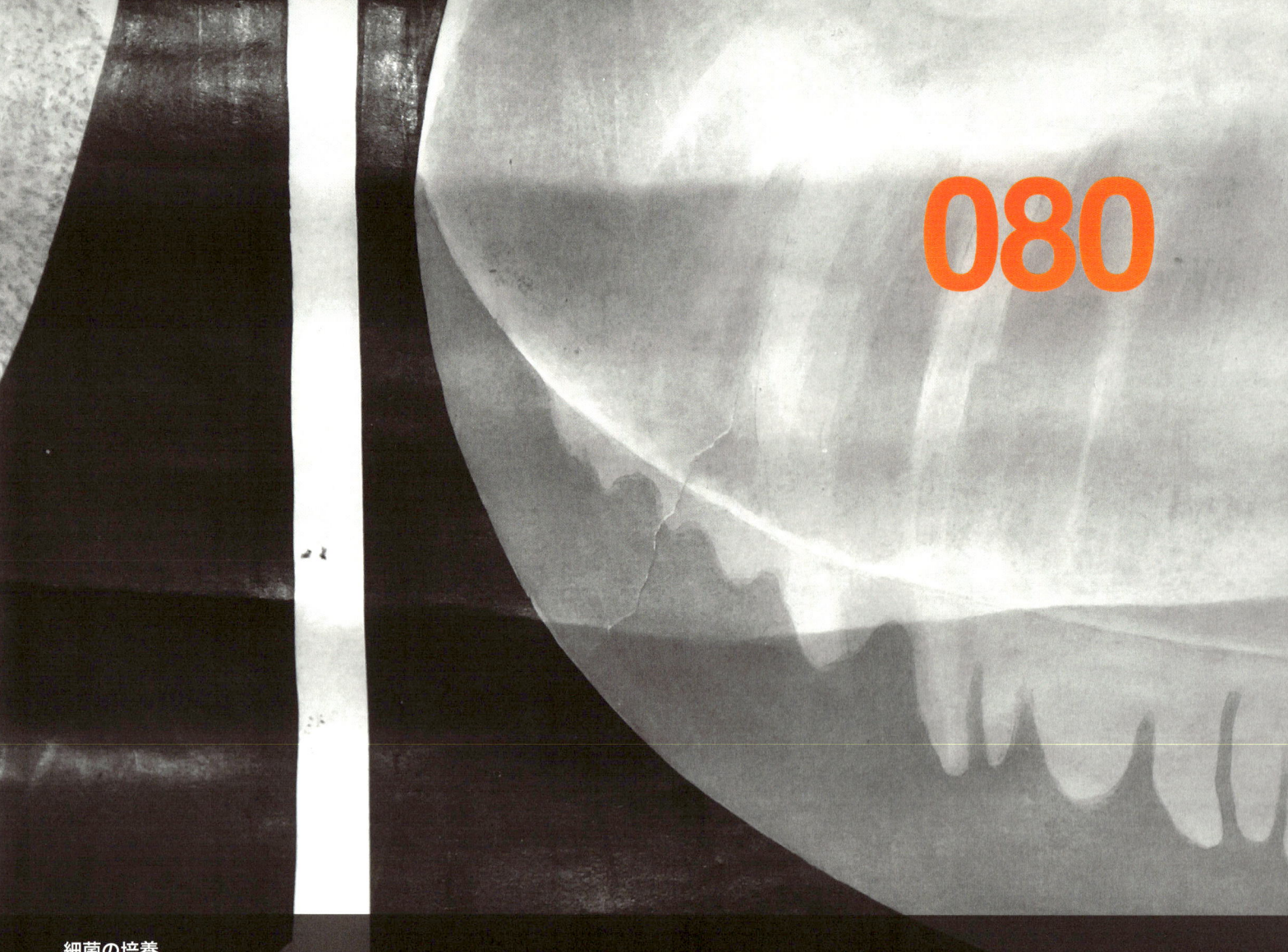

080

細菌の培養
明治中期／軸装掛図、水彩画／全長940、本紙縦804、横1094、軸長1119／東京大学総合研究博物館研究部所蔵

細菌という肉眼では見えない敵と戦ってきた細菌学の歴史を表す資料。ジフテリア病変部位から菌を培養すると、病原菌であるジフテリア菌以外に連鎖球菌等との混合感染もあり、菌分離・同定が困難なことも多い。左図(A)はジフテリア菌と連鎖球菌が血清を含んだ培地上にコロニー(菌の塊)を形成しているところを光に透かして見たもの。右図(B)はブイヨン培地を入れたフラスコ内でジフテリア菌を培養している場面を表したものである。現在、2種(ジフテリア・破傷風)および3種混合ワクチン(前記2種および百日咳)が普及しているため、ジフテリア菌の感染によるジフテリア罹患者は、2001年以降、国内で確認されていない。しかし、現在でも海外からもち込まれる恐れがあり、感染力や罹患した場合の重篤性からみて危険性が高い感染症である2類感染症に指定されている。ジフテリアの致死率は5から10パーセント程度であるが、1884年にフリードリッヒ・レフレル(1852–1915)が菌の純粋培養に成功した頃は、死亡率が40パーセントにものぼり、一刻も早い治療法の確立が望まれていた。ジフテリアの治療、予防に大きく貢献したのは本邦の北里柴三郎(1853–1931)である。

The Culture of Bacilli
Mid-Meiji period / Wall chart on scroll, watercolor / L940; Illustration: L804, W1094; Scroll: L1119 / Research Department, UMUT

Document presenting the history of bacteriology, a discipline which has been fighting with an enemy invisible to the naked eye. When culturing bacteria from a lesion affected by diphtheria, streptococci appear along with the pathogen diphtheria bacilli, and the mixed infection complicates the isolation and identification of bacteria. The illustration on the left (A) shows a colony of diphtheria bacilli and streptococci propagating on a serum plate. It is slightly enlarged due to transmitted light. On the right, the illustration (B) shows diphtheria bacilli propagating in bouillon as a culture medium, within a flask. Currently, with the generalization of combined vaccination for diphtheria, pertussis and tetanus, there is no recorded case of a contamination by the diphtheria bacillus in Japan since 2001. However, as the risk of bringing bacteria from abroad remains, and given its infectious capacity and the seriousness of the affection, it is still classified as a second-class infectious disease. The lethality of diphtheria is rated at only 5 to 10%, but when in 1884 Friedrich Loeffler (1852 – 1915) succeeded in the pure culture of the bacillus, the mortality rate rose to 40%, necessitating an immediate treatment method. Shibasaburo Kitazato (1853 – 1931) greatly contributed to the treatment and prevention of diphtheria.

A   **B**

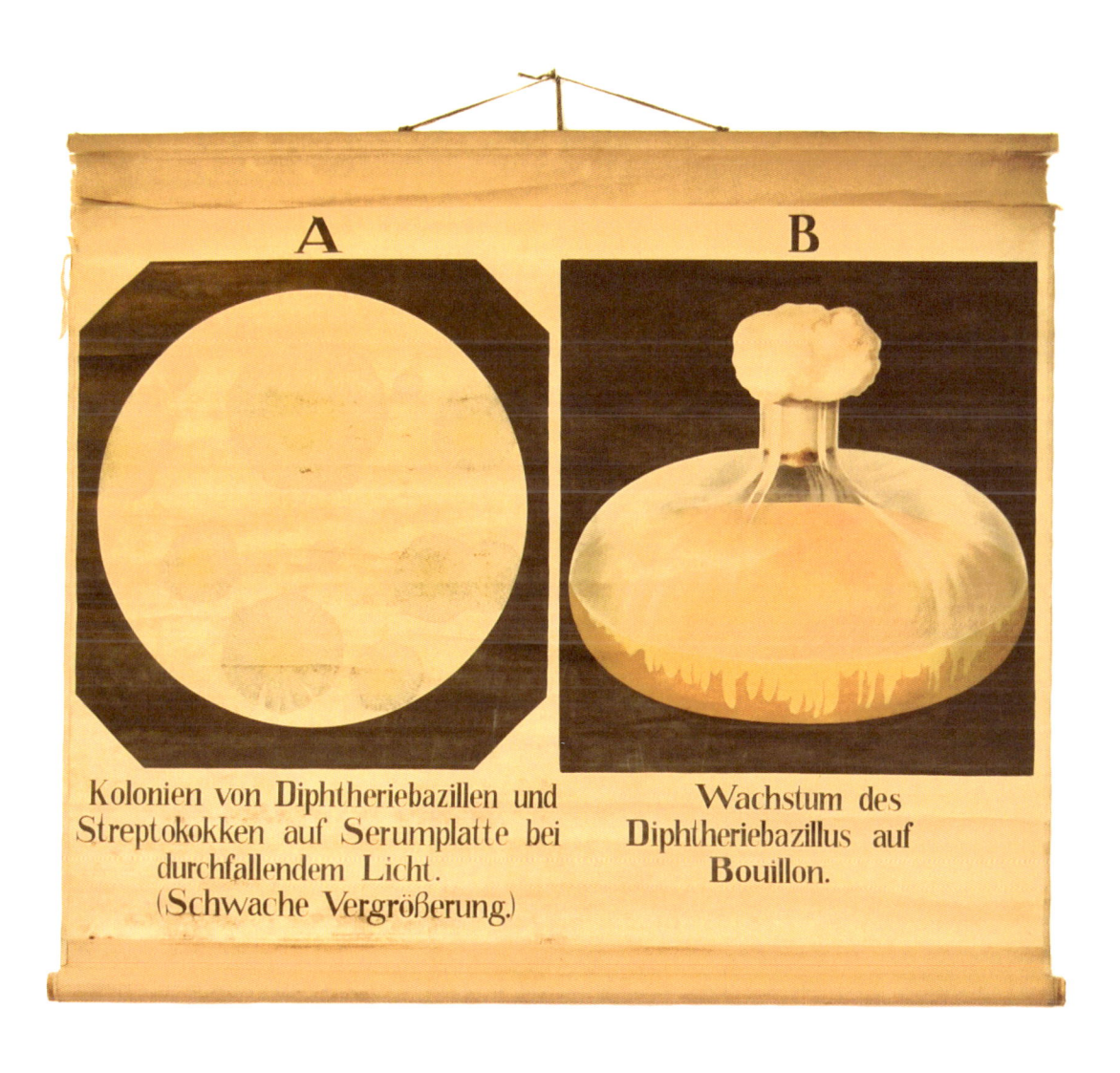

Kolonien von Diphtheriebazillen und Streptokokken auf Serumplatte bei durchfallendem Licht. (Schwache Vergrößerung.)

Wachstum des Diphtheriebazillus auf Bouillon.

082

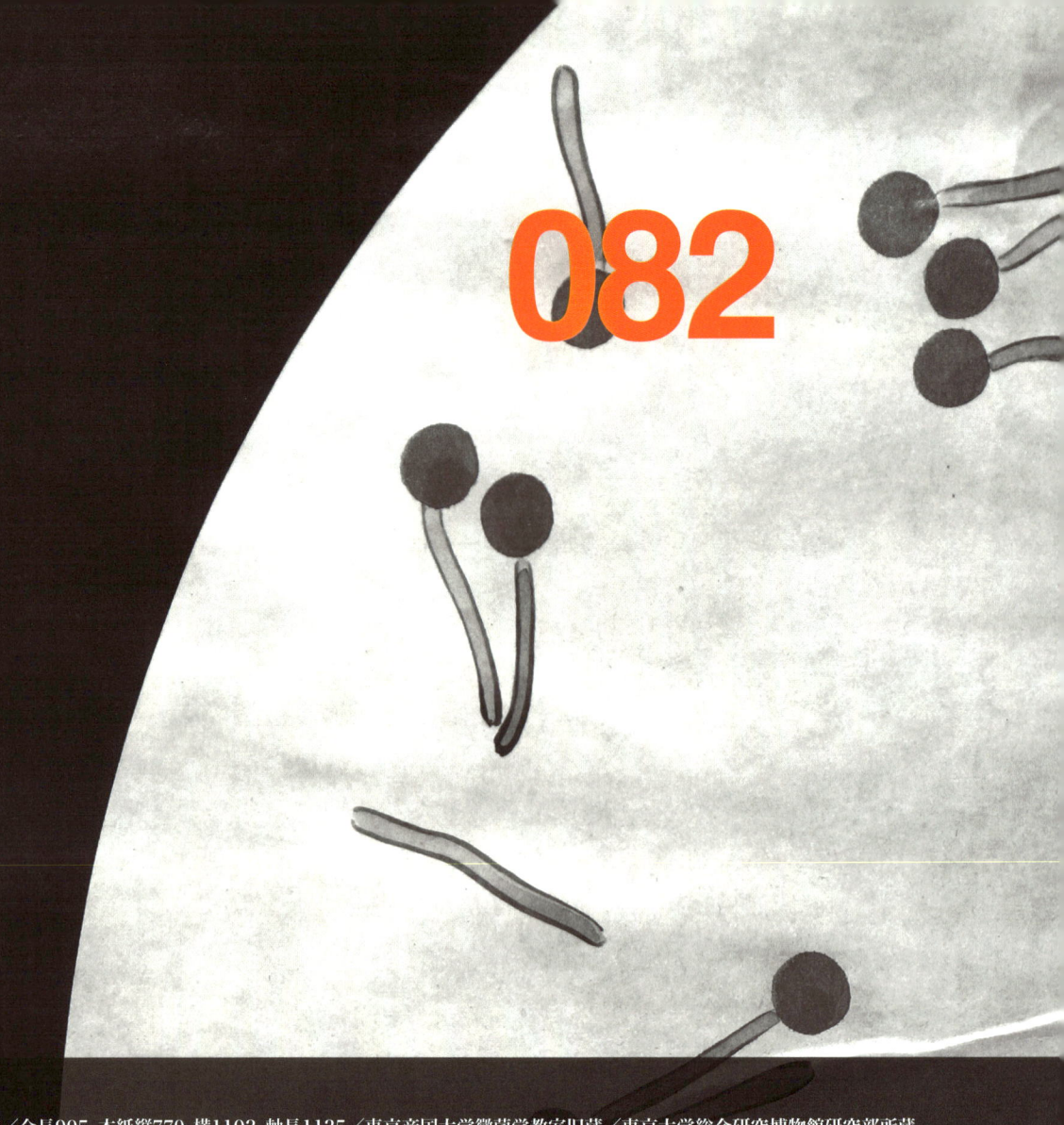

破傷風菌

明治中期／軸装掛図、水彩画／全長905、本紙縦770、横1103、軸長1135／東京帝国大学黴菌学教室旧蔵／東京大学総合研究博物館研究部所蔵

破傷風の病原菌である破傷風菌は芽胞のかたちで土壌中にも広く分布しており、傷口から体内に入ると発芽、増殖、毒素を産生し、痙攣や呼吸困難を生じさせる。日本における1950年の罹患者は1千9百名超、致死率は80パーセント超と、重篤な病気であった。しかし、1968年に3種混合ワクチンの定期予防接種が開始され、罹患者、致死率ともに減少し、現在では年間数名から百名程度の罹患者数で、致死率も20から50パーセント程度となっている。これに大きく貢献したのが北里柴三郎(1853–1931)である。北里は1889年に、当時不可能とされていた破傷風菌の純粋培養を世界で初めて成功させ、翌年には破傷風菌の抗毒素(現在で言う「抗体」)を発見、引き続き血清療法という画期的な手法を開発した。これはジフテリアの血清療法にも繋がった。本図は破傷風菌を純粋培養したものを2種の方法を用いて染色したものである。

Tetanus Bacillum

Mid-Meiji period / Wall chart on scroll, watercolor / L905; Illustration: L770, W1103; Scroll: L1135 / Former collection of the Laboratory of Bacteriology, Imperial University of Tokyo / Research Department, UMUT

The tetanus bacillum, pathogen of tetanus, is widely spread in the soil. When introduced into the body through a wound, it grows, propagates and produces toxins, causing convulsions and dyspnea. In 1950, victims in Japan exceeded 1900 cases with a death rate of more than 80%, making tetanus a serious disease. However, with the implementation of combined vaccination in 1968, the number of victims as well as the lethality of tetanus fell, and the number of victims now amounts to 50 to 100 per year, with a death rate of 20 to 50%. Shibasaburo Kitazato (1853 – 1931) greatly contributed to this. In 1889, he succeeded in the pure culture of tetanus bacilli, which was then considered impossible, and the following year, he discovered the antitoxin (or antibody, as we would say today) to tetanus, before developing the revolutionary method of serotherapy. This eventually led to the adoption of serotherapy for diphtheria. The present illustration shows two types of coloration for tetanus bacilli grown in pure culture.

Fig. 1. Fig. 2.

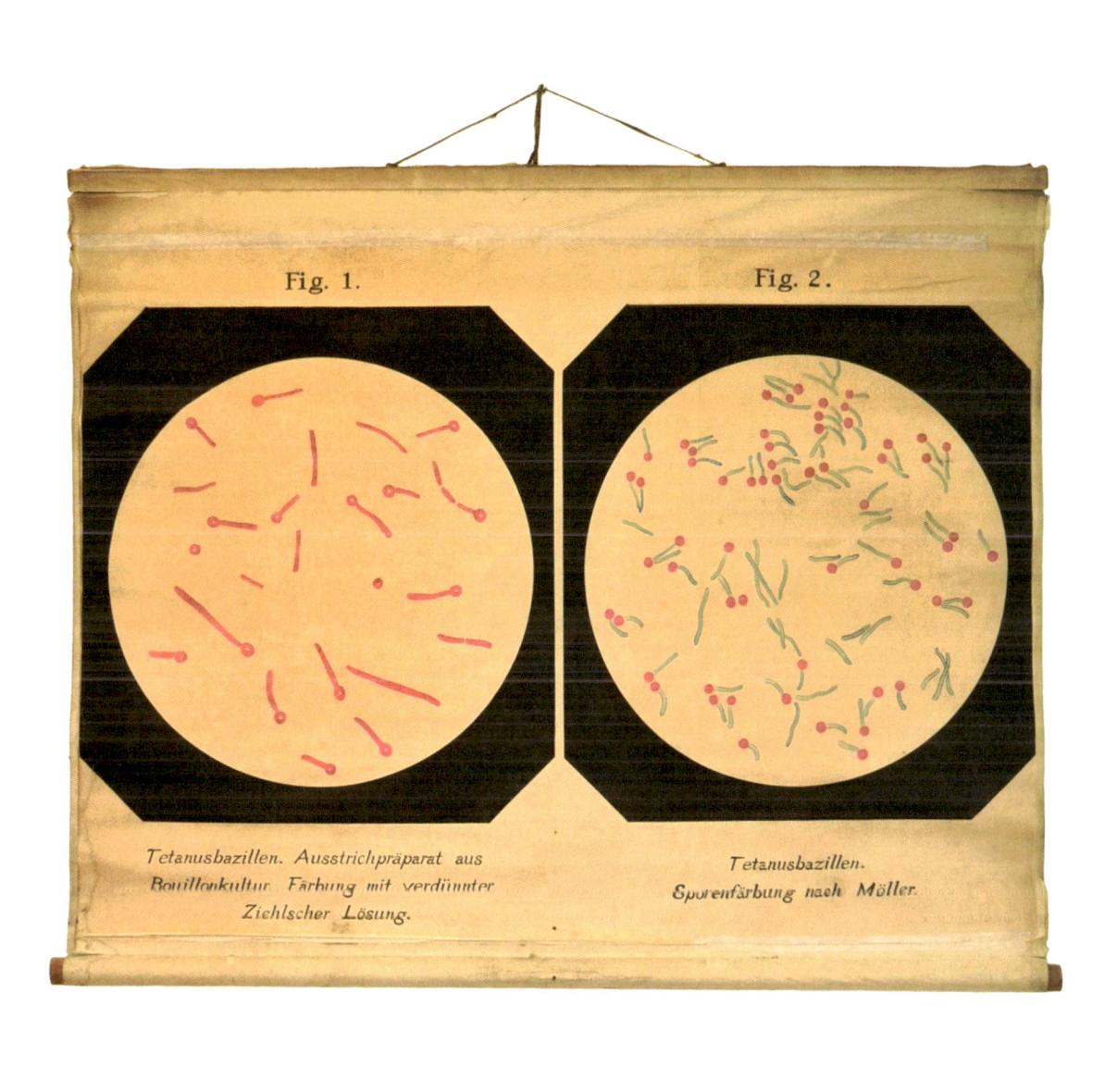

Tetanusbazillen. Ausstrichpräparat aus Bouillonkultur. Färbung mit verdünnter Ziehlscher Lösung.

Tetanusbazillen. Sporenfärbung nach Möller.

084

腸管を支配する自律神経
明治中期／軸装掛図、水彩画／全長2170、本紙縦1778、横945、軸長965／東京大学医学部旧蔵／東京大学総合研究博物館研究部所蔵

人間の身体には、意識せずとも体内をつねに一定の状態に保とうとする様々な仕組みが備わっている。その仕組みのひとつに、神経（自律神経系）による調節がある。暑ければ発汗し、走れば脈拍が速くなる。腸管の収縮運動も同様の作用による。腸管運動はゆったりと休んでいる時に盛んになるよう、自然と調整されている。本図は腸管運動を調整する自律神経系の神経の走行である。大きく分けて自律神経系には、人間の活動時によく働く交感神経系と、休息時によく働く副交感神経系がある。赤が交感神経系を、青が副交感神経系を表す。

Autonomic Nerves Controlling the Digestive Tract
Mid-Meiji period / Wall chart on scroll, watercolor / L2170; Illustration: L1778, W945; Scroll: L965 / Former collection of the Faculty of Medicine, The University of Tokyo / Research Department, UMUT

The human body is driven by various unconscious mechanisms working to maintain a stable internal condition. One of such mechanisms is the regulation by nerves (and the autonomic nervous system). It provokes perspiration under the effect of heat, and a pulse acceleration when running. The contractions of the digestive tract also follow such a mechanism. The digestive tract is naturally regulated so as to become active when the body is resting. The present illustration shows the repartition of autonomic nerves controlling the digestive tract. Roughly speaking, the autonomic nervous system can be divided in two types: the sympathetic nervous system especially working during man's active state, and the parasympathetic nervous system working when man is at rest. The former is shown in red, and the latter in blue.

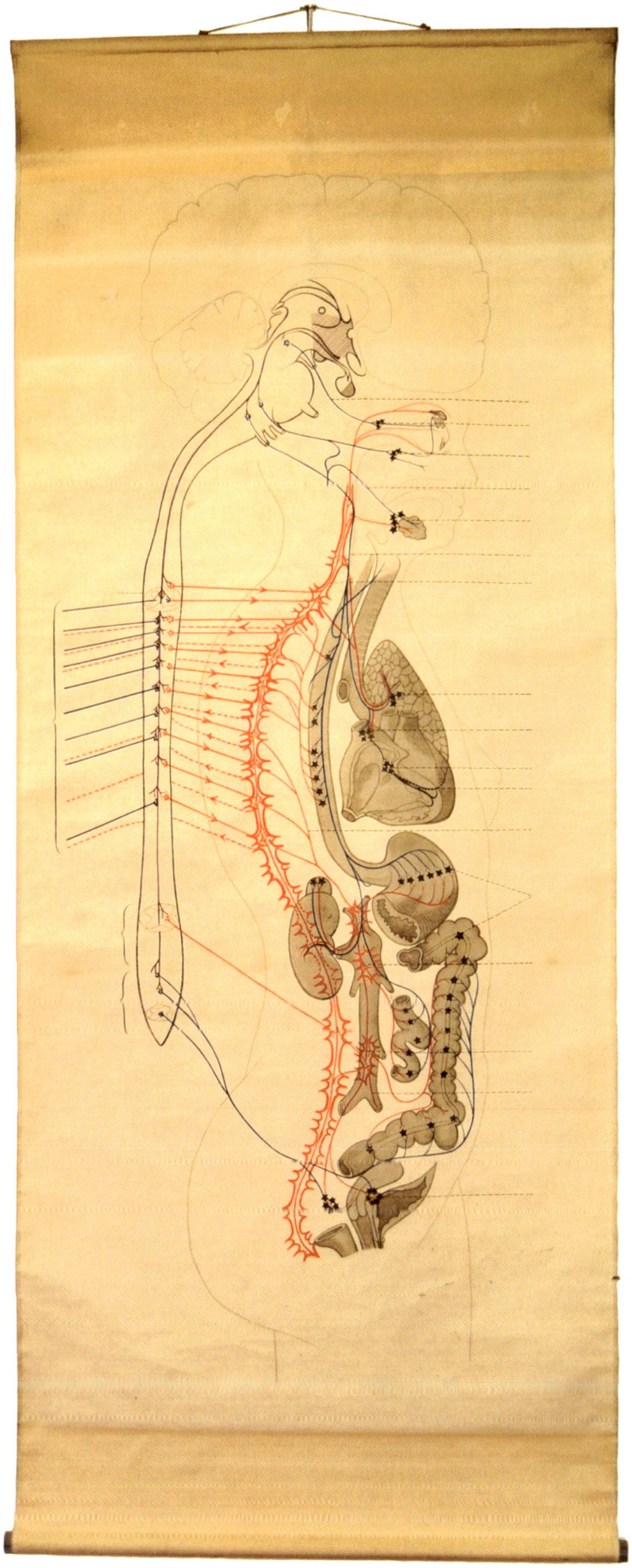

086

動脈の神経支配
明治中期／軸装掛図、水彩画／全長2080、本紙縦1690、横890、軸長912／東京大学総合研究博物館研究部所蔵

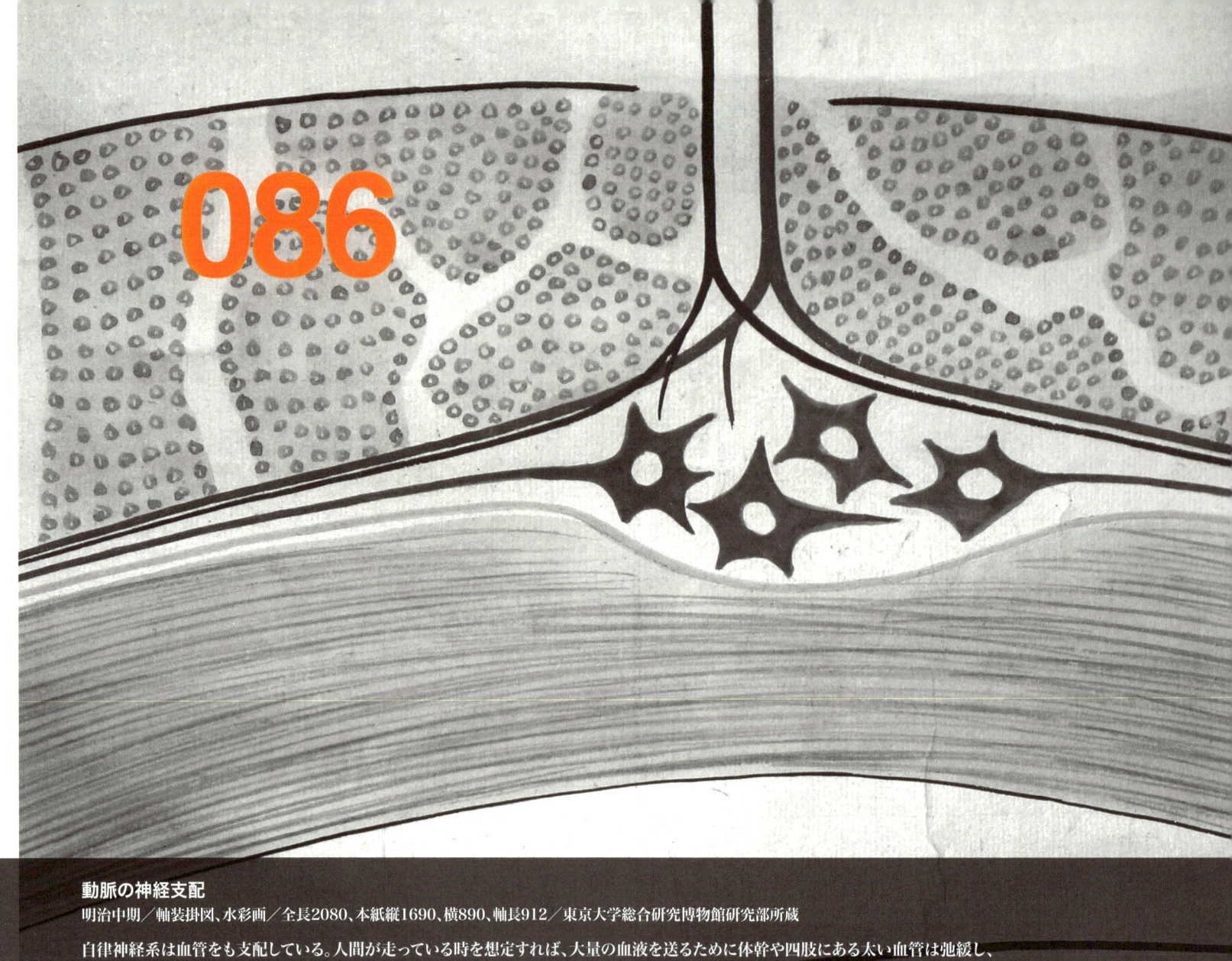

自律神経系は血管をも支配している。人間が走っている時を想定すれば、大量の血液を送るために体幹や四肢にある太い血管は弛緩し、使用されない末梢の細い血管は収縮する。これは意識せずとも自然に働く交感神経系の作用による。その血管運動（収縮や弛緩）の中枢は脳の脳幹と呼ばれる部分に存在する。本図は血管運動の中枢からの支配を描いたものである。

Nervous Control of the Arteries
Mid-Meiji period / Wall chart on scroll, watercolor / L2080; Illustration: L1690, W890; Scroll: L912 / Research Department, UMUT

The autonomic nervous system also controls blood vessels. For instance, when man is running, thick vessels running in the trunk and the limbs relax in order to send important volumes of blood, whereas unused thin veins in the periphery contract. This is due to the natural activity of the sympathetic nervous system. The contraction and relaxation activity of blood vessels is centered around the brain stem, located within the brain. The present illustration shows the control of blood vessels from this crucial point.

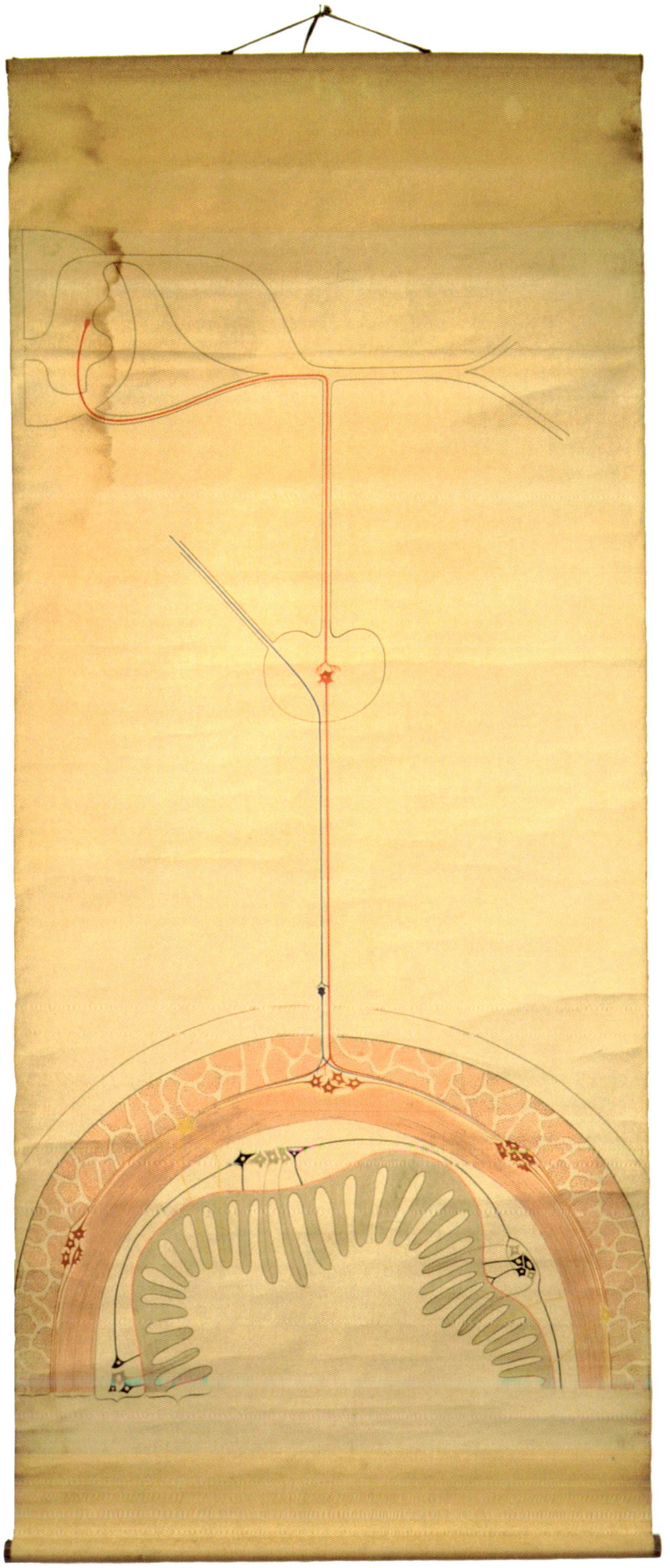

カエル解剖図（頸部の神経を示す）
明治中期／軸装掛図、水彩画／全長1310、本紙縦955、横839、軸長869／東京大学総合研究博物館研究部所蔵

エドゥアルト・フリードリヒ・ヴィルヘルム・ヴェーバー（1806–1871）はカエルの迷走神経に電気刺激を加えて心臓の働きが抑制されることを発見し、1845年にナポリで開かれた学会で報告した。これは神経系の作用によって自律運動が抑制される世界初の観察例であった。カエルの迷走神経の位置と、その方法を示したのが本図である。心臓もまた自律神経系に支配されており、休息時には自然とわれわれの脈拍も遅くなっている。これは全身で必要とされる酸素と栄養が減少し、その結果、それらを運ぶ循環血液量は少なくて済むからである。この調整も無意識のうちに行われているが、これは副交感神経系のひとつである迷走神経の働きによる。

Anatomical Chart of Frog
Mid-Meiji period / Wall chart on scroll, watercolor / L1310; Illustration: L955, W839; Scroll: L869 / Research Department, UMUT

Eduard Friedrich Wilhelm Weber (1806 – 1871) discovered that by electrically stimulating a frog's vagus nerve, its heart movements could be controlled. He reported his discovery in a convention held in 1845 in Naples. It was the first observation case of an autonomic activity being controlled through an intervention on the nervous system. The present illustration shows the location of the frog's vagus nerve, and the method employed. The heart is also controlled by the autonomic nervous system, and our pulse slows down when we are at rest. This is due to the decrease in oxygen and nutrients necessitated by the whole body, which in turn allows for a reduction in the amount of circulating blood carrying them. This process is also controlled unconsciously, and it is the activity of the vagus nerve, which belongs to the parasympathetic nervous system.

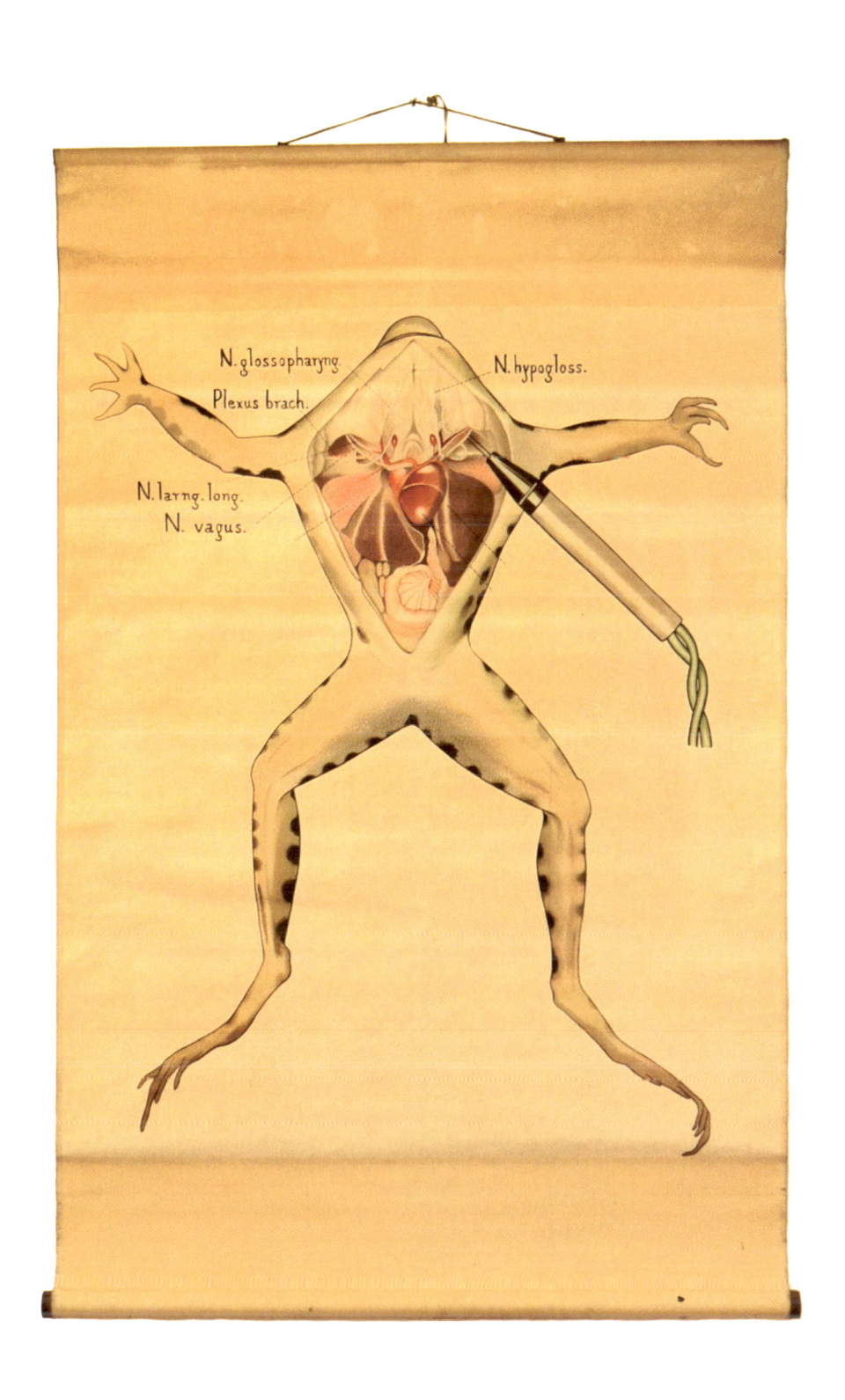

N. glossopharyng.   N. hypogloss.
Plexus brach.

N. laryng. long.
N. vagus.

大脳解剖図(横断面)
明治中期／軸装掛図、印刷に墨書／全長1075、本紙縦1035、横775、軸長791／東京大学総合研究博物館研究部所蔵

脳は均質ではない。神経細胞体が集まっている部分があり、そのような部分は他の脳の部位に比べ色が濃く、解剖学的に見ても周囲から区別できる。これが「核」と呼ばれる部位であり、それぞれ機能的な特徴を有している。本図は大脳の水平断面(図の左と右では異なった高さで切った様子が合わさっている)を示し、解剖学的に特徴のある脳の各部位がその名前とともに示されている。人体の構造と機能を知ることが医学の基礎であり、その構造を明らかにする学問が解剖学である。

Anatomical Chart of Cerebrum
Mid-Meiji period / Wall chart on scroll, ink on print / L1075; Illustration: L1035, W775; Scroll: L791 / Research Department, UMUT

The brain is not homogeneous. Parts concentrating nerve cells are darker in color than other parts of the brain, and the distinction can also be made from an anatomical point of view. This part is called "gray matter," and has characteristic functions. The present illustration shows a horizontal cross-section of the cerebrum (the left and right parts illustrating the cross-section at different levels of the brain), with the names of each anatomically significant part of the brain. The base of medicine consists in knowing the structure and functions of the human body, and anatomy is the discipline clarifying its structure.

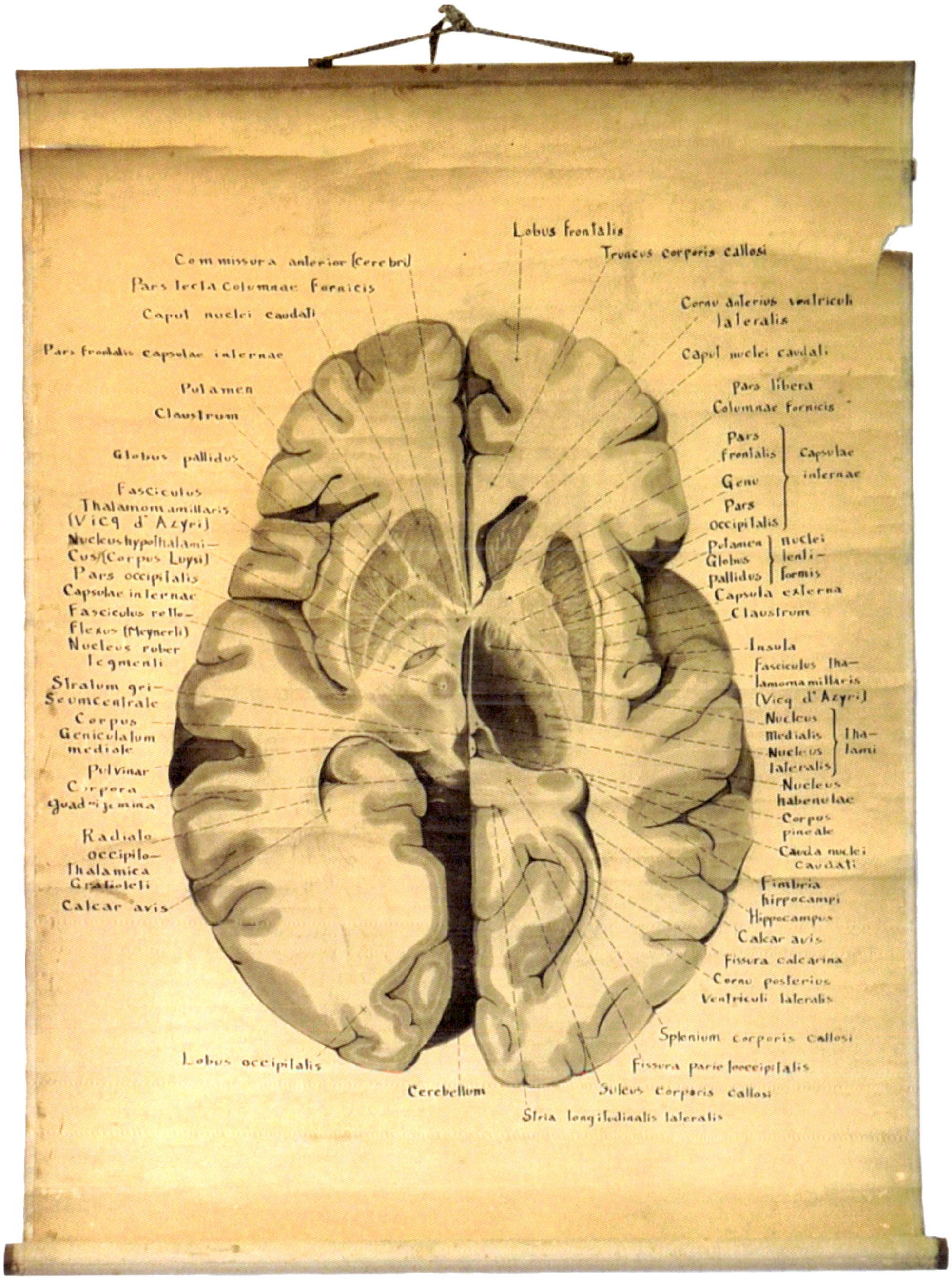
Lobus frontalis
Truncus corporis callosi
Commissura anterior (cerebri)
Pars tecta columnae fornicis
Caput nuclei caudati
Pars frontalis capsulae internae
Putamen
Claustrum
Globus pallidus
Fasciculus Thalamomamillaris (Vicq d' Azyri)
Nucleus hypothalamicus (Corpus Luysi)
Pars occipitalis Capsulae internae
Fasciculus retroflexus (Meynerti)
Nucleus ruber tegmenti
Stratum griseum centrale
Corpus Geniculatum mediale
Pulvinar
Corpora Quadrigemina
Radiatio occipito-thalamica Gratioleti
Calcar avis
Lobus occipitalis
Cerebellum
Stria longitudinalis lateralis
Cornu anterius ventriculi lateralis
Caput nuclei caudati
Pars libera Columnae fornicis
Pars frontalis
Genu
Pars occipitalis
Capsulae internae
Putamen
Globus pallidus
nuclei lentiformis
Capsula externa
Claustrum
Insula
Fasciculus thalamomamillaris (Vicq d' Azyri)
Nucleus medialis
Nucleus lateralis
Thalami
Nucleus habenulae
Corpus pineale
Cauda nuclei caudati
Fimbria hippocampi
Hippocampus
Calcar avis
Fissura calcarina
Cornu posterius Ventriculi lateralis
Splenium corporis callosi
Fissura parieto-occipitalis
Sulcus corporis callosi

092

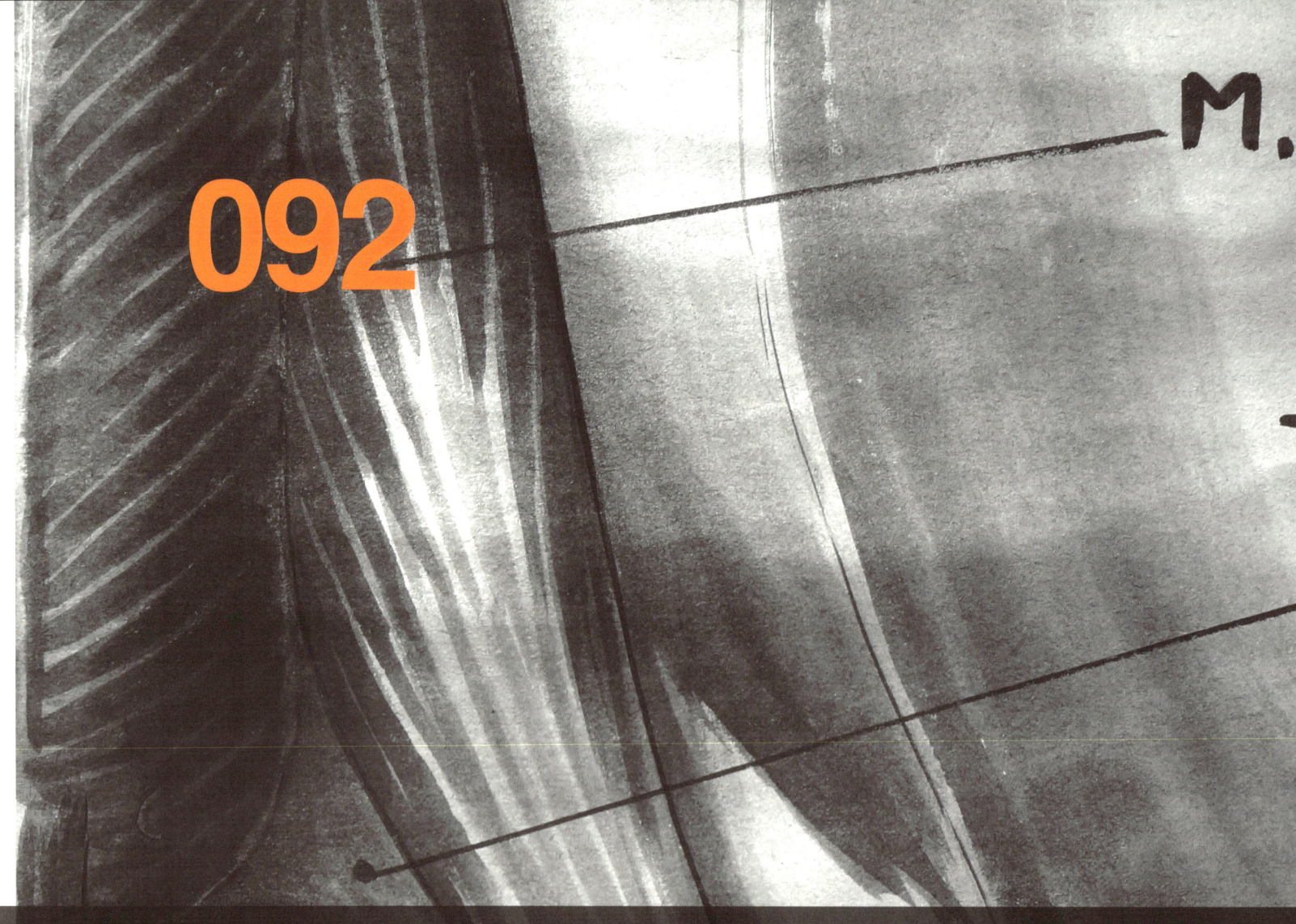

男性の会陰部解剖図
明治中期／軸装掛図、印刷に彩色／全長1210、本紙縦1068、横777、軸長794／東京大学総合研究博物館研究部所蔵

会陰とは本来、肛門と外陰部の間の小さい領域のみを指した言葉であるが、骨盤からの出口全体を示す広い意味で使われることが多い。すなわち、恥骨結合の下縁、左右の大腿、そして臀部で囲まれる菱形の領域の事である。この部位を解剖し、スケッチしたのが本図である。この部位にある筋は大きく分けて2種類存在する。ひとつが外陰部の筋、もうひとつが腸の末端の筋である。これらをまとめて会陰筋と呼ぶ。前者に5つ、後者に3つの筋が存在する。本図は男性の解剖図であるが、女性との差が外観的に認められるのは、外陰部の5つの筋のうち1つの筋肉、すなわち球海綿体筋のみである。

Anatomical Chart of Male Perineum
Mid-Meiji period / Wall chart on scroll, coloring on print / L1210; Illustration: L1068, W777; Scroll: L794 / Research Department, UMUT

Initially, the perineum designated the small area between the anus and the external genitalia, but it is now frequently used to signify more generally the zone around the orifice of the pelvis, in other words the diamond-shaped zone constituted by the lower part of the pubic joint, both thighs and the rear. The present illustration is an anatomical sketch of that zone. Roughly, two types of nerves are found in this part: those of the external genitalia, and those of the extremity of the intestine. The present illustration is that of a male, but the only externally visible difference with the female is one of the five muscles of the external genitalia, that is the bulbocavernosus muscle.

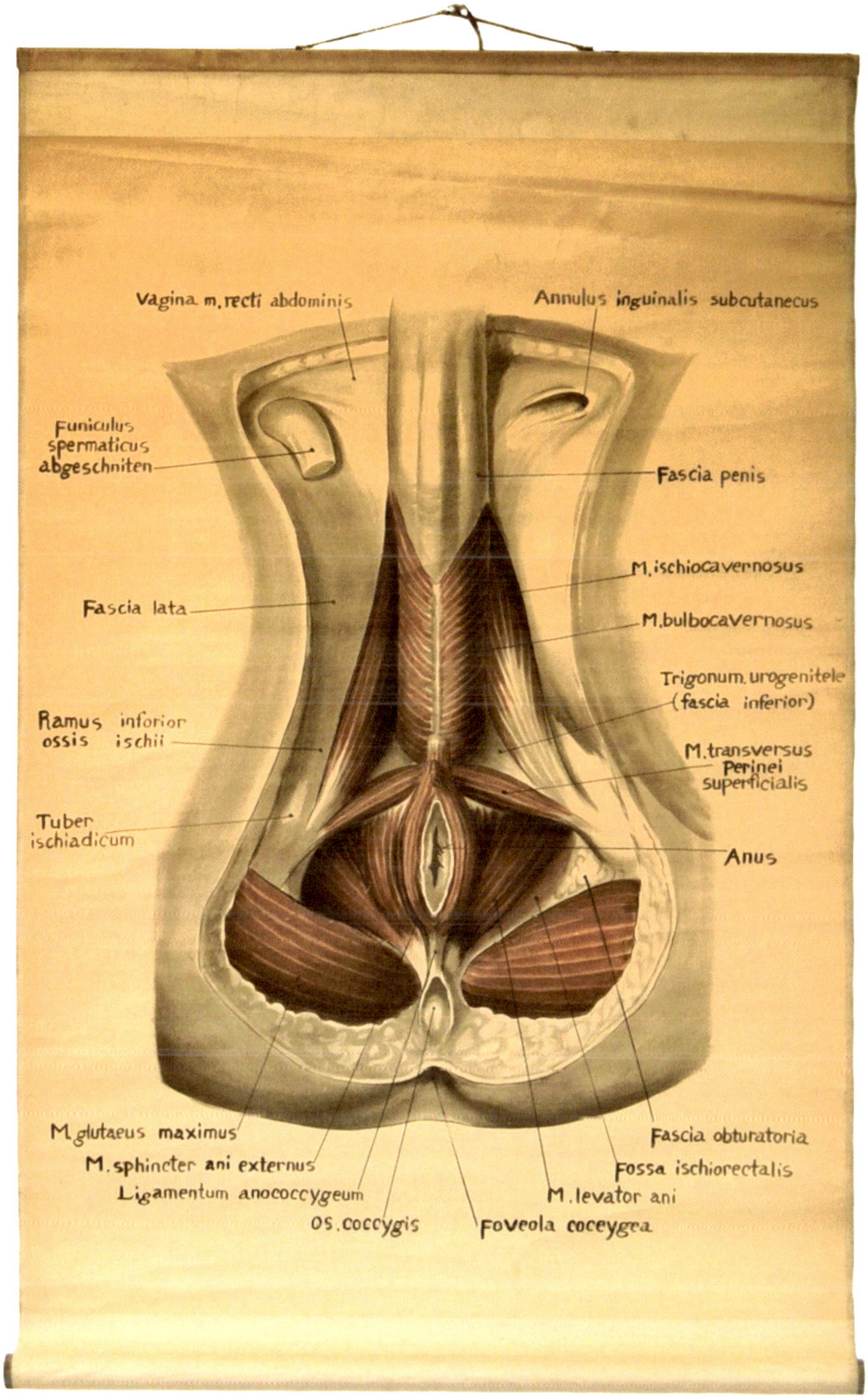
Vagina m. recti abdominis
Annulus inguinalis subcutanecus
Funiculus spermaticus abgeschniten
Fascia penis
M. ischiocavernosus
Fascia lata
M. bulbocavernosus
Trigonum urogenitele (fascia inferior)
Ramus inforior ossis ischii
M. transversus Perinei superficialis
Tuber ischiadicum
Anus
M. glutaeus maximus
Fascia obturatoria
M. sphincter ani externus
Fossa ischiorectalis
Ligamentum anococcygeum
M. levator ani
Os. coccygis
Foveola coceygea

094

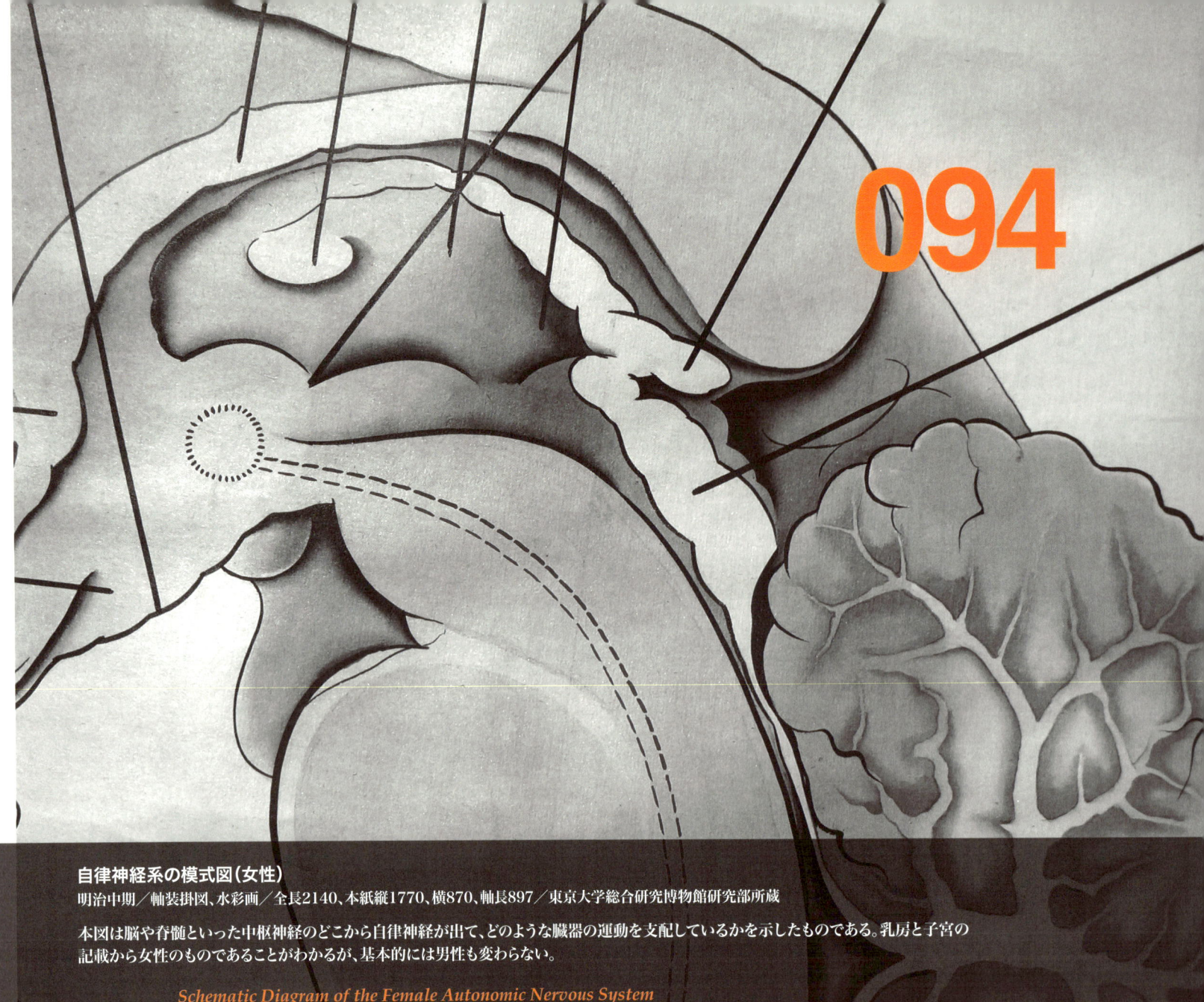

自律神経系の模式図（女性）
明治中期／軸装掛図、水彩画／全長2140、本紙縦1770、横870、軸長897／東京大学総合研究博物館研究部所蔵

本図は脳や脊髄といった中枢神経のどこから自律神経が出て、どのような臓器の運動を支配しているかを示したものである。乳房と子宮の記載から女性のものであることがわかるが、基本的には男性も変わらない。

Schematic Diagram of the Female Autonomic Nervous System
Mid-Meiji period / Wall chart on scroll, watercolor / L2140; Illustration: L1770, W870; Scroll: L897 / Research Department, UMUT

The present illustration shows the parts of the central nerves from which the autonomic nerves emanate, and which organs they control. Mentions of the bosom and of the uterus indicate that this is a female, but there is no fundamental difference with the male.

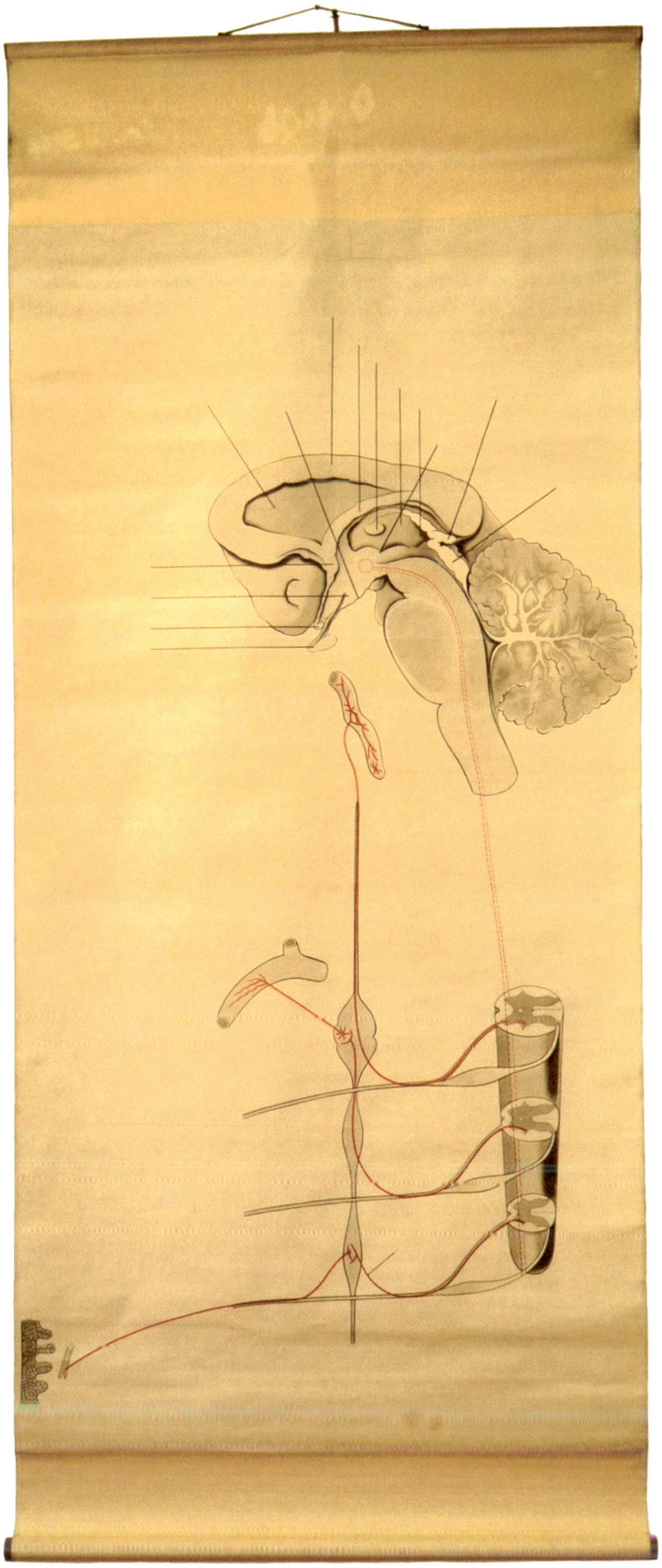

096

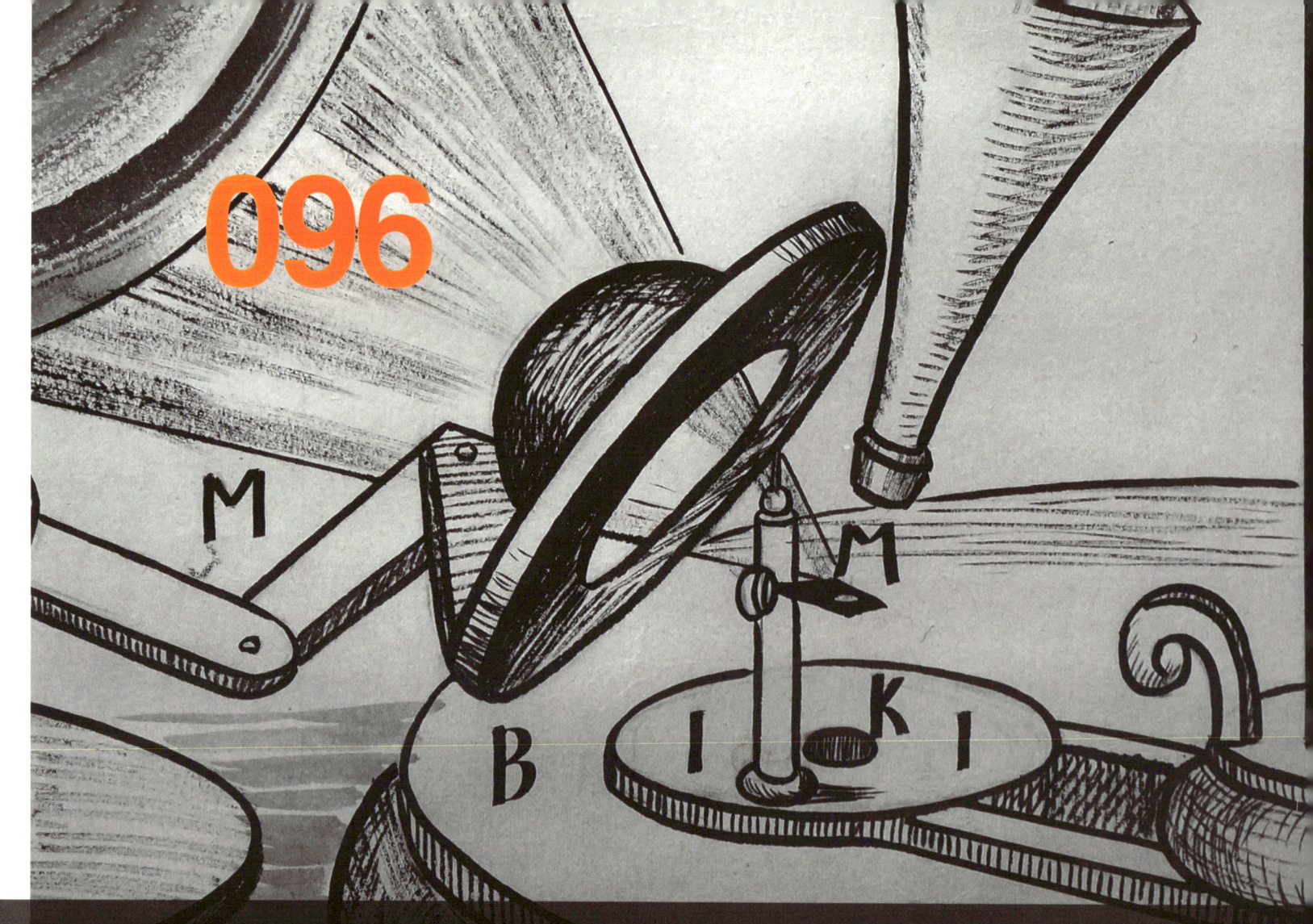

顕微鏡
明治中期／軸装掛図、水彩画／全長1020、本紙縦785、横818、軸長878／東京大学総合研究博物館研究部所蔵

顕微鏡でなければ観察できない細胞、その「細胞」という言葉を生みだしたのはロバート・フック（1635–1703）であった。彼が使っていた顕微鏡はクリストファー・コックという人物が作製したものだが、光を集めて観察し易くするなど、その設計はフック自身が行ったものだと言われる。本図はフックの著書『ミクログラフィア』（1665年）に描かれている顕微鏡装置図の一部を抜粋したもので、まさに彼はこの顕微鏡を使用して同著を執筆した。同著中では、装置の説明に引き続き、詳細に同顕微鏡の詳細が語られている。『ミクログラフィア』発刊当初、望遠鏡により宇宙が、そして顕微鏡により小さな世界を観察することができるようになっていたが、顕微鏡はまだ珍しい器械にすぎなかった。しかし、彼は身の回りのあらゆるものを顕微鏡で観察し、自然の造形物の緻密な構造に驚嘆した。フックは顕微鏡で観察して見たものをただ単に描いただけでなく、鋭い洞察力や想像力をもって科学史に多大な影響を与えた。われわれの身体を構成している細胞、その内部にもさらに微細な構造があり、現在の解剖学はこのような微細構造ならびにその機能を明らかにしようとしている。人体もまた壮大な宇宙と言うことができる。

Microscope
Mid-Meiji period / Wall chart on scroll, watercolor / L1020; Illustration: L785, W818; Scroll: L878 / Research Department, UMUT

It is Robert Hooke (1635 – 1703) who forged the word "cell" to designate these entities invisible to the naked eye. His microscope was made by a certain Christopher Cocks, but it is said that Hooke himself designed it so as to facilitate observation by concentrating light. The present illustration is an extract of the diagram of the microscopic device drawn in Hooke's *Micrographia* (1665), the device Hooke used to write his book. The publication includes an explanation as well as numerous details on this device. At the time of the publication of *Micrographia*, it was already possible to observe the cosmos with the telescope and the realm of the infinitesimal through the microscope, but the latter was still nothing more than a rare instrument. However, Hooke observed everything around him with the microscope, and was astonished at the minute structure of all natural creation. Not only did Hooke draw what he saw through the microscope, but through his acute sense of observation and imagination, he also held a considerable influence on the history of science. The cells structuring our body themselves have a finer structure, and current anatomy attempts to clarify such cellular structure and functions. We can thus state that the human body is also a gigantic universe.

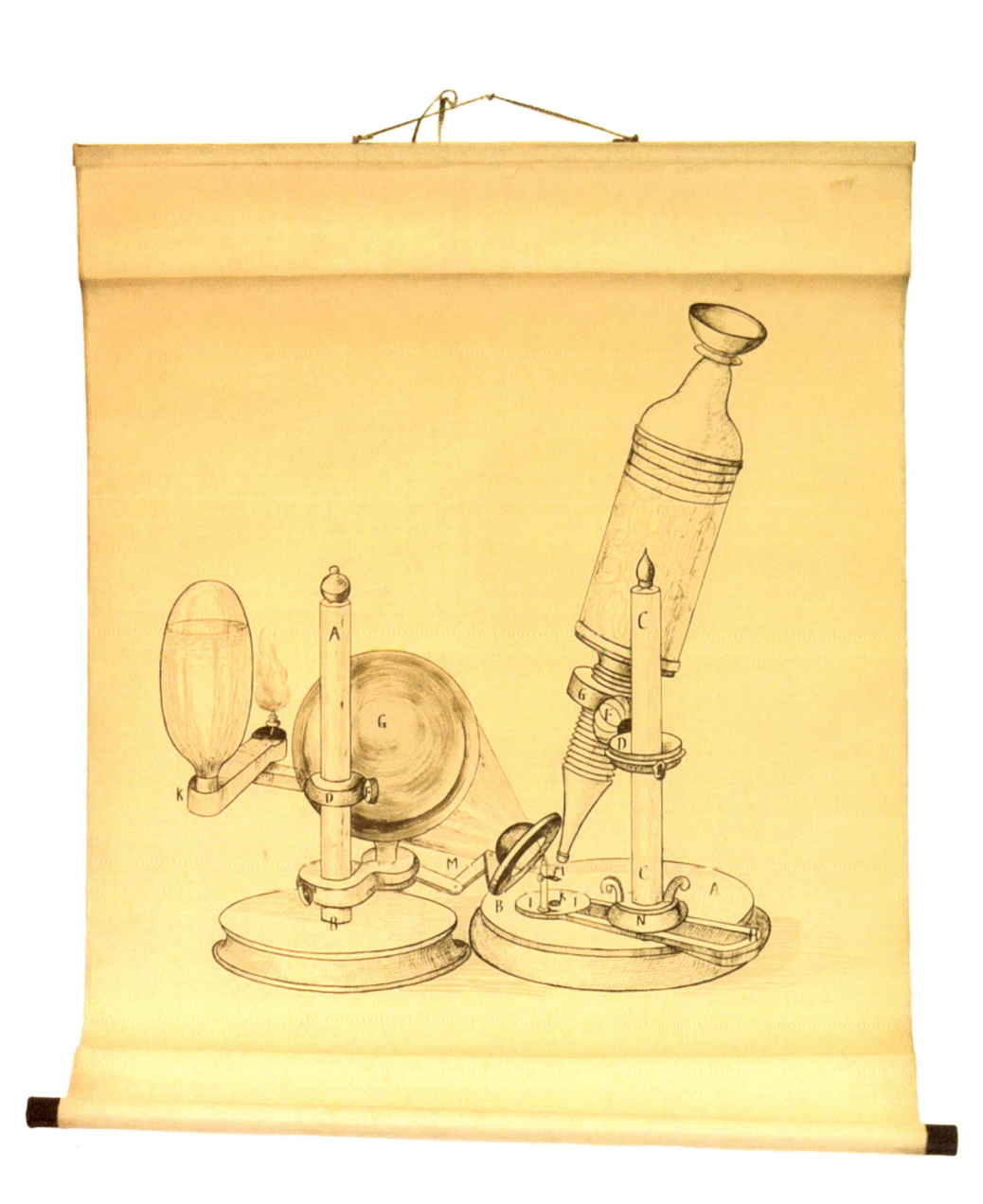

098

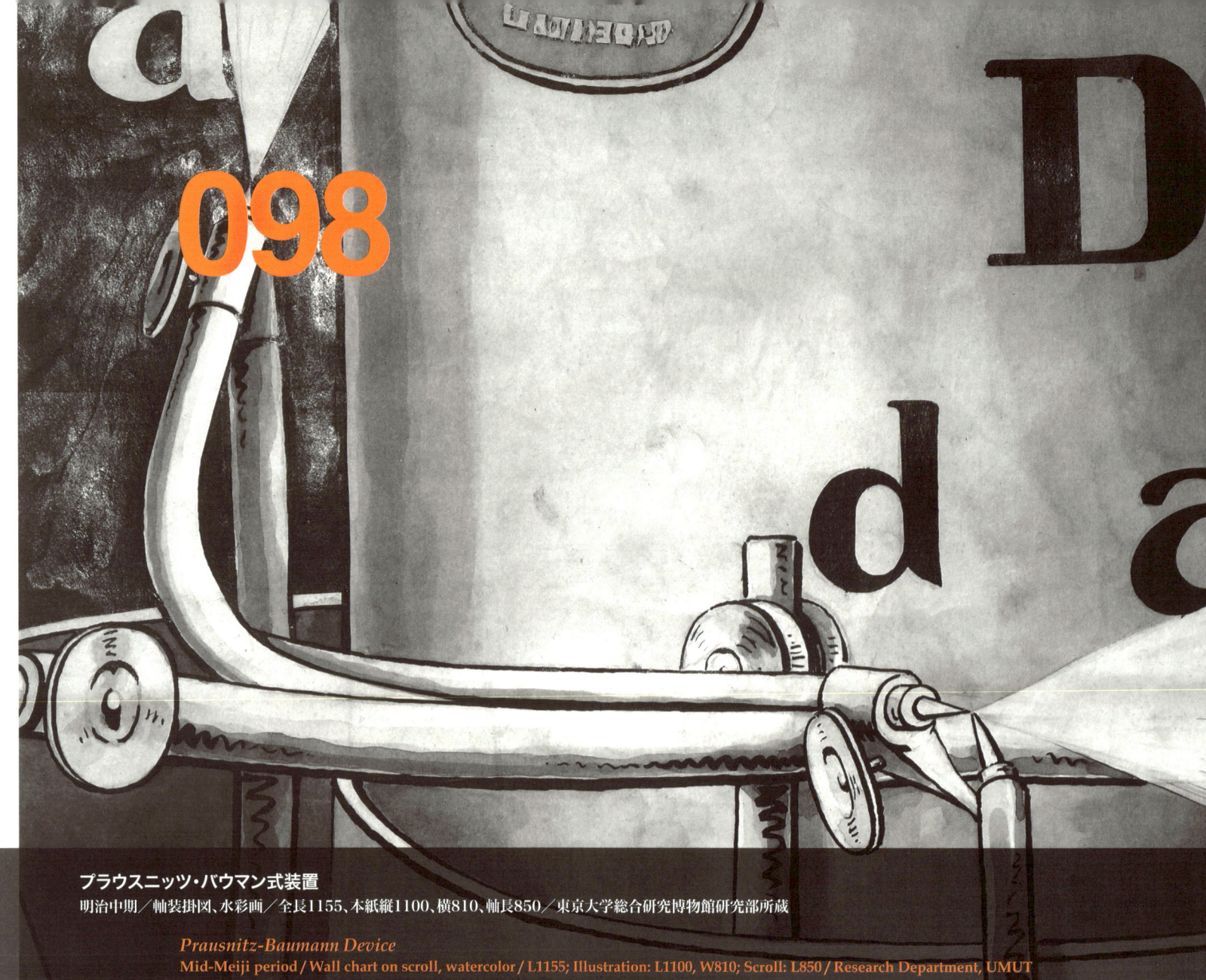

プラウスニッツ・バウマン式装置
明治中期／軸装掛図、水彩画／全長1155、本紙縦1100、横810、軸長850／東京大学総合研究博物館研究部所蔵

Prausnitz-Baumann Device
Mid-Meiji period / Wall chart on scroll, watercolor / L1155; Illustration: L1100, W810; Scroll: L850 / Research Department, UMUT

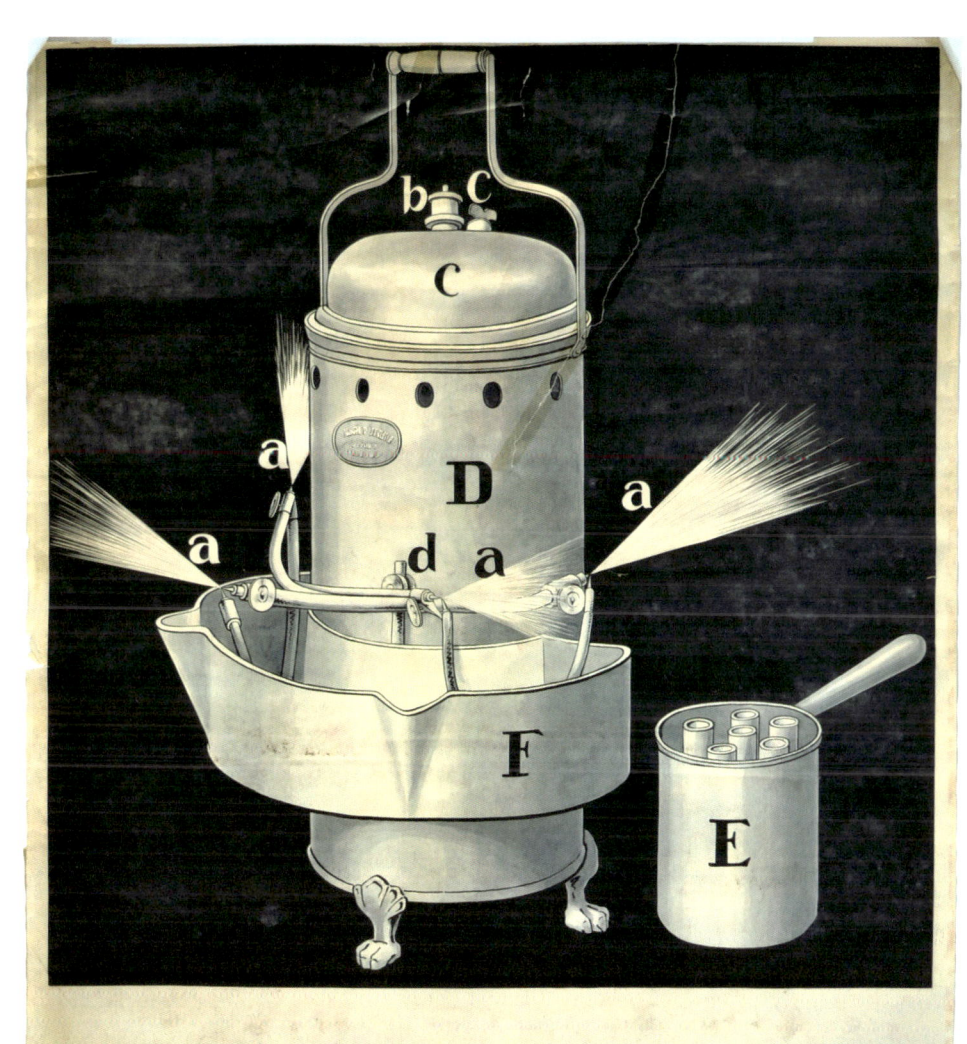

Prausnitz-Baumann'scher Apparat.

Private collection

個人コレクション

102

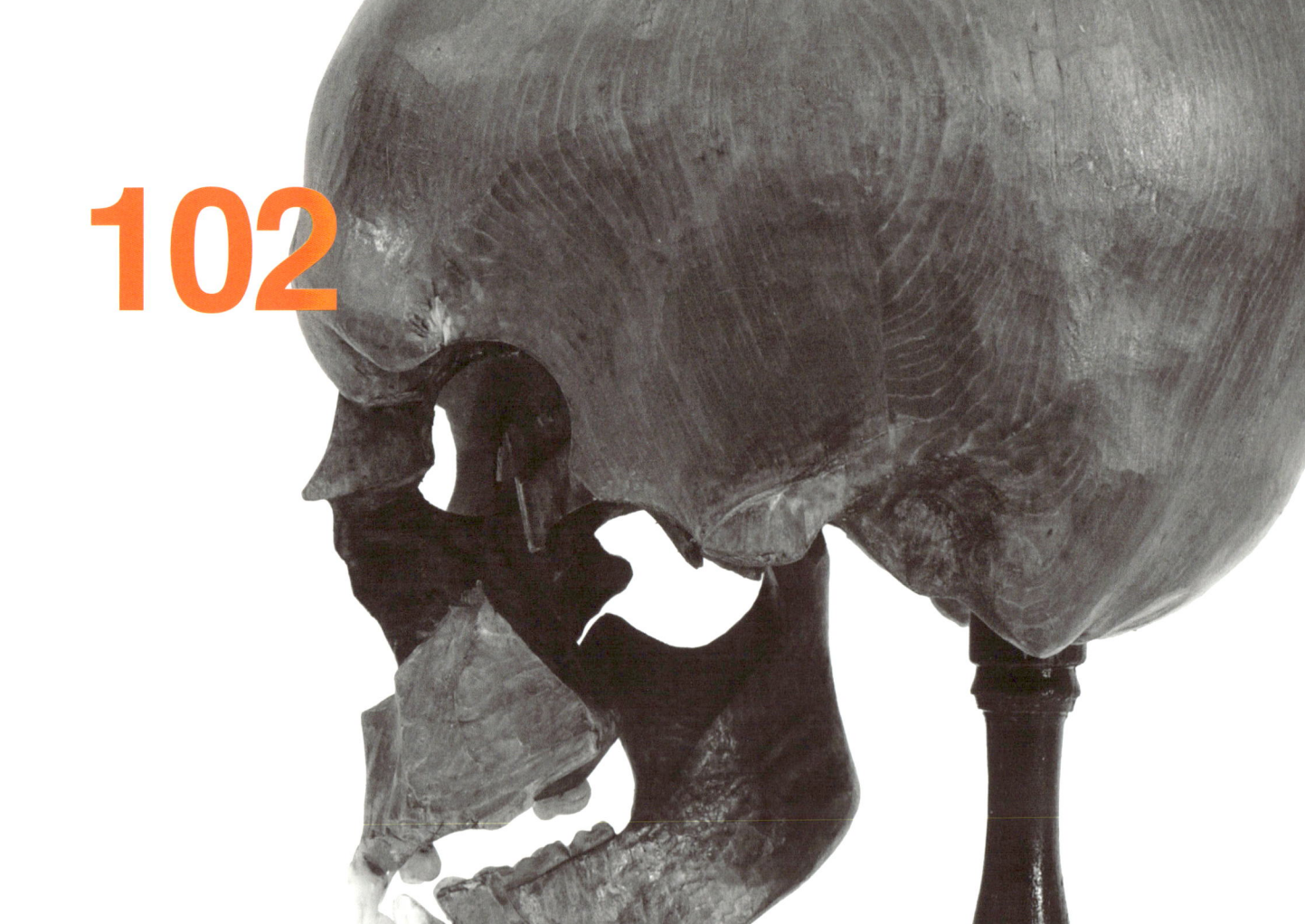

人頭蓋
平成24（2012）年／菊池敏正制作／檜に漆、彩色、セラミクス／縦210、横210、高300／個人蔵

鎌倉時代人の頭骨を基に、模刻したもの。檜材を寄せ木して、彫刻を施すという伝統的な仏像制作技術による。ただし、歯の部分には、質感を再現するため、現代素材のセラミクスが使われている。

Human Skull
2012 / Made by Toshimasa Kikuchi / Lacquer on Japanese cypress, coloring, ceramics / L210, W210, H300 / Private collection

Wood carving of a skull from the Kamakura period, based on the traditional Buddhist sculpting technique of mounting Japanese cypress and carving it. In order to render best their texture, the teeth are now made of ceramics.

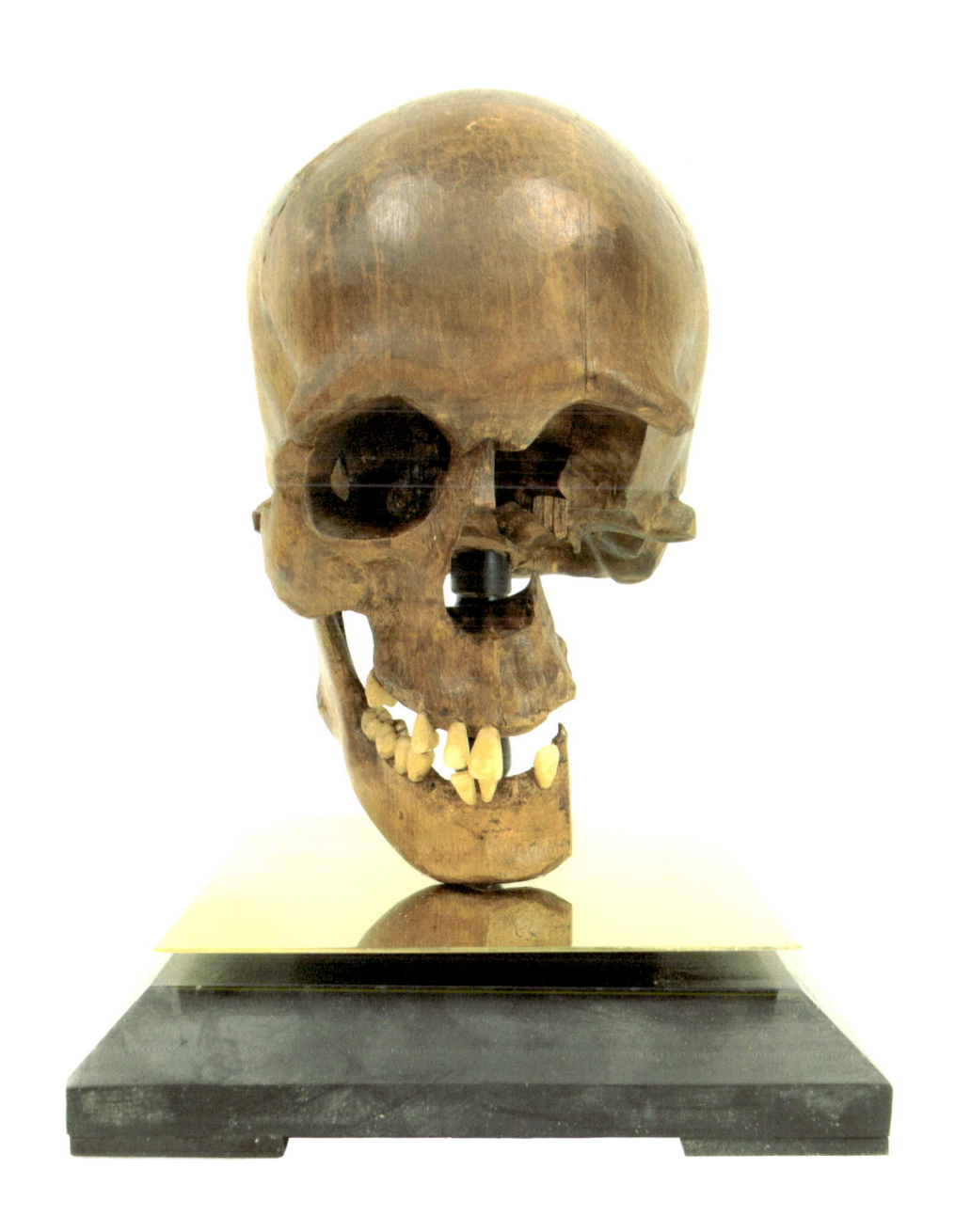

104

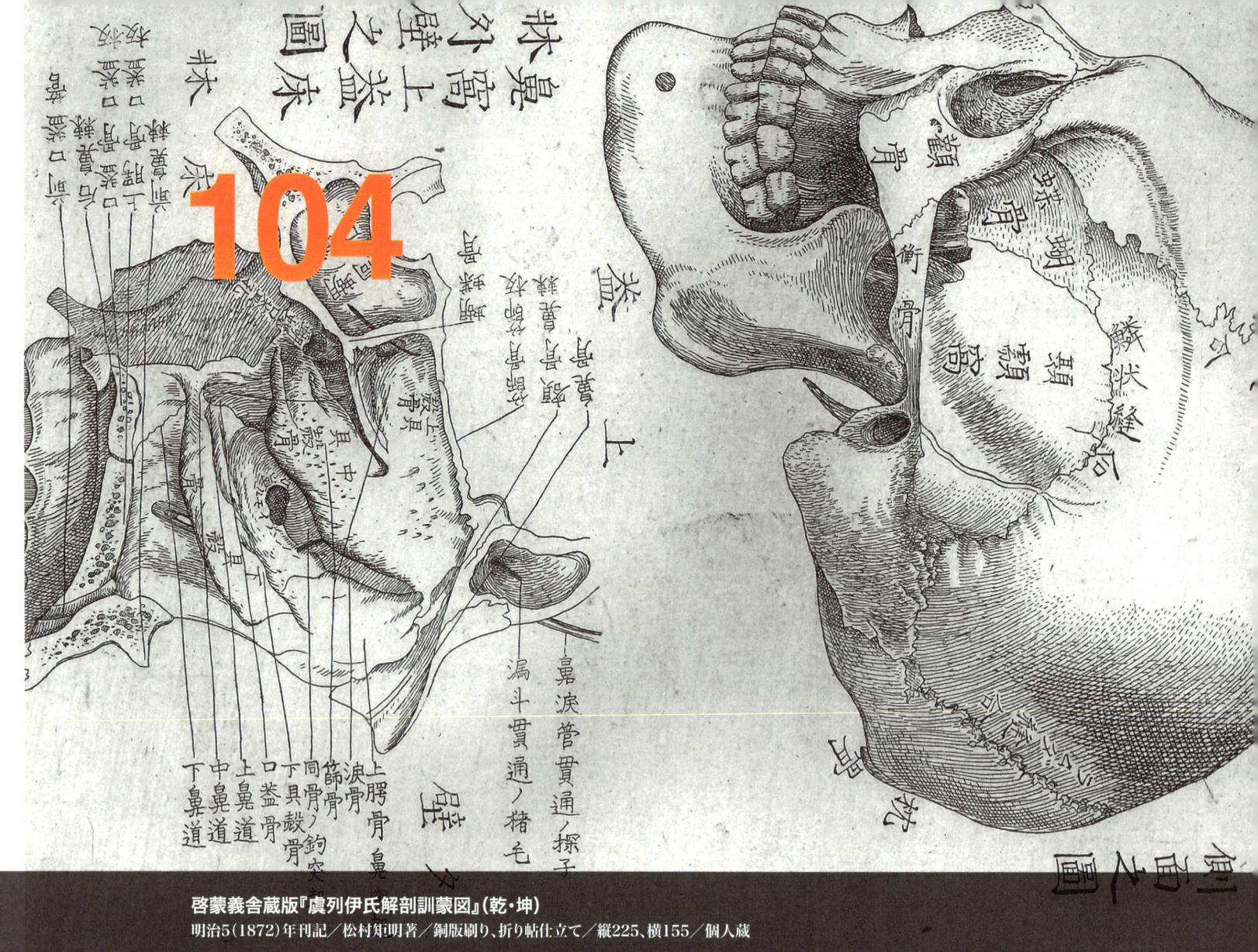

啓蒙義舎蔵版『虞列伊氏解剖訓蒙図』（乾・坤）
明治5（1872）年刊記／松村矩明著／銅版刷り、折り帖仕立て／縦225、横155／個人蔵

イギリスの解剖学者ヘンリー・グレイ（1827-1861）の『人体解剖学』を底本とする。1852年に25歳の若さで王立協会のフェローの栄誉を受けたグレイは、1861年に34歳の若さで病死しているが、「グレイの解剖学」と通称された主著の評判は高かったようである。事実、同書の初版は1858年で、1860年には版を重ねている。原本に掲げられた363点の図版を制作したのは、クレイの友人の外科医で、父親が画家であったことから解剖図の制作にも長けていたヘンリー・ヴァンダイク・カーター（1831-1897）である。明治時代になると解剖図譜にも、当然、これまで以上の精度が求められるようになった。幕末の啓蒙医松村矩明（1842-1877）の翻訳出版になる『解剖訓蒙』（1872年）は図版の評判が悪かったため、英人グレイの『人体解剖学』第5版の図譜を銅版翻刻した本図譜乾坤2冊を出版することで、その不備を補ったという。松村は、敦賀出身の蘭方医で、明治元（1868）年に大坂医学校校長となった。

Illustrated Encyclopedia of Gray's Anatomy in Two Volumes, Keimogisha Version
Published in 1872 / Written by Noriaki Matsumura / Copperplate printing, accordion binding / L225, W155 / Private collection

Based on the *Anatomy of the Human Body* of British anatomist Henry Gray (1827 – 1861). Gray, elected Fellow of the Royal Society at the early age of 25, died of a disease in 1861 at the age of 34. Nevertheless, his main publication, commonly entitled *Gray's Anatomy*, had a high reputation. In fact, the first edition dates back to 1858, but it was already reprinted in 1860. The author of the original edition's 363 illustrations was Henry Vandyke Carter (1831 – 1897), Gray's friend and a surgeon who also excelled in anatomical drawing, his father being a painter. In the Meiji period, a higher degree of precision was naturally required for anatomical illustrations. Noriaki Matsumura (1842 – 1877), a preeminent physician from the end of the Edo period, had published a translation under the title of *Encyclopedia of Anatomy* (1872), but its illustrations were criticized. To make up for it, the two volumes of the present publication were published, with a copperplate reprint of the illustrations of the fifth edition of Gray's *Anatomy of the Human Body*. Matsumura was a Dutch-style physician native of Tsuruga, who became director of the Osaka School of Medicine in 1868.

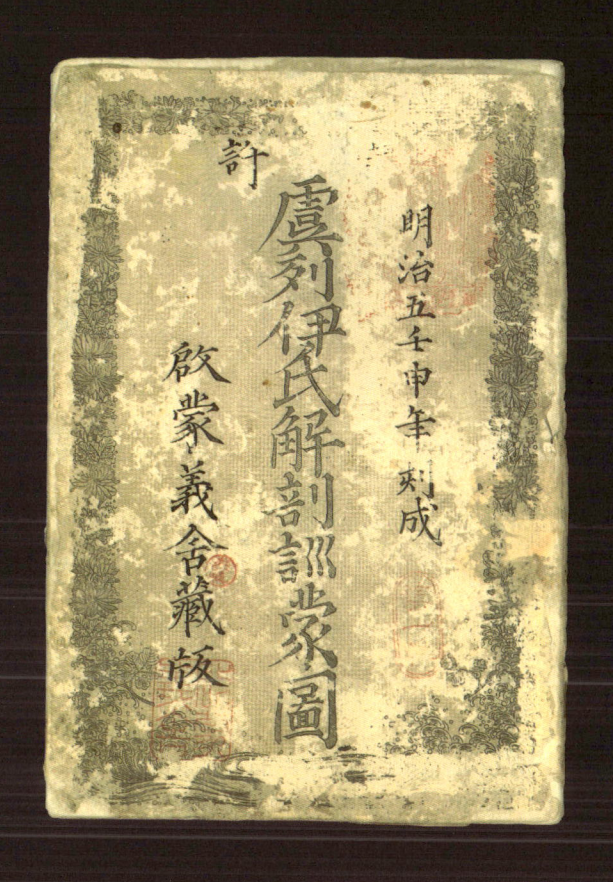

軎列伊氏解剖諭蒙圖

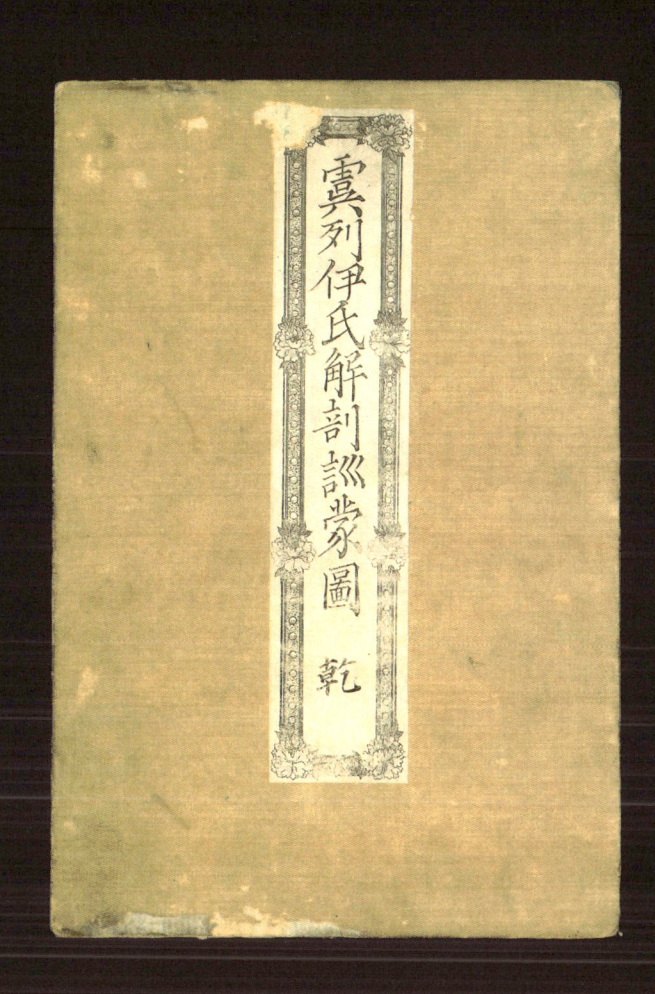

表紙：
- 明治五壬申年刻成　虞列伊氏解剖諭蒙圖　啓蒙義舎藏版
- 雲列伊氏解剖諭蒙圖　乾

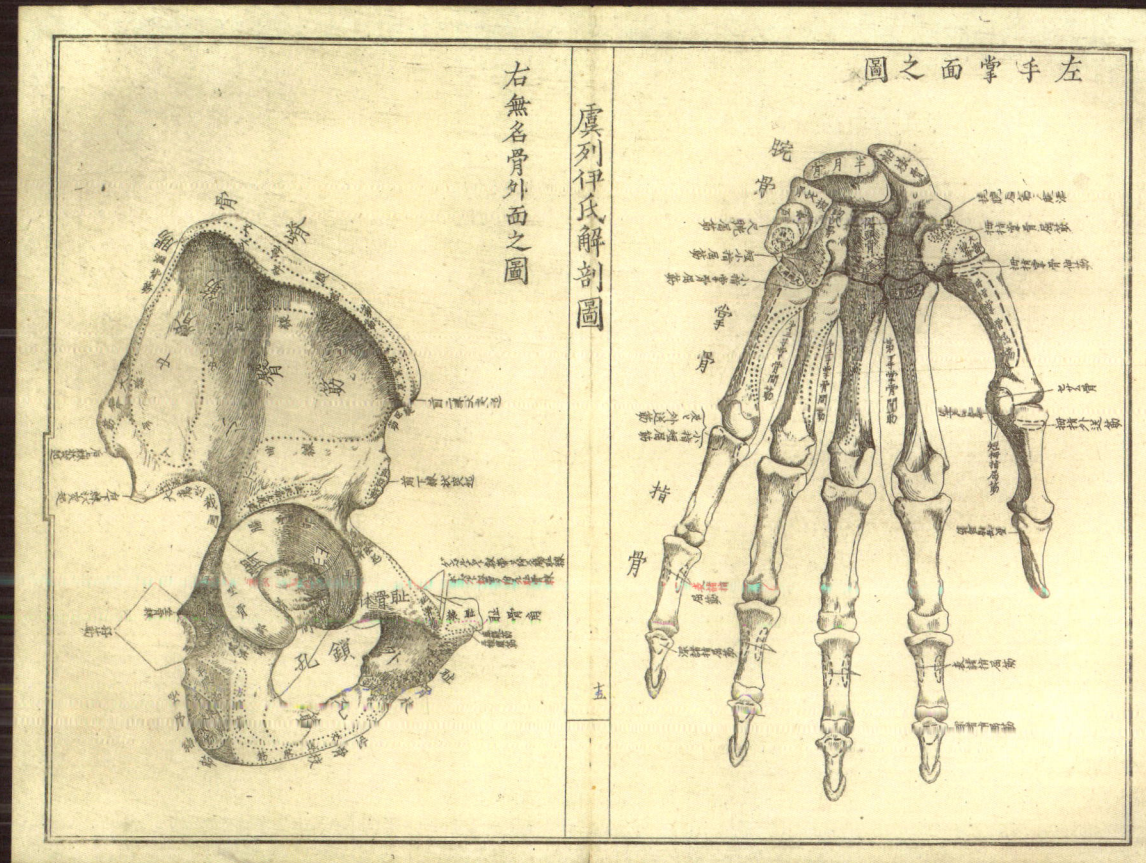

左手掌面之圖

腕骨　掌骨　指骨

右無名骨外面之圖

虞列伊氏解剖圖

106

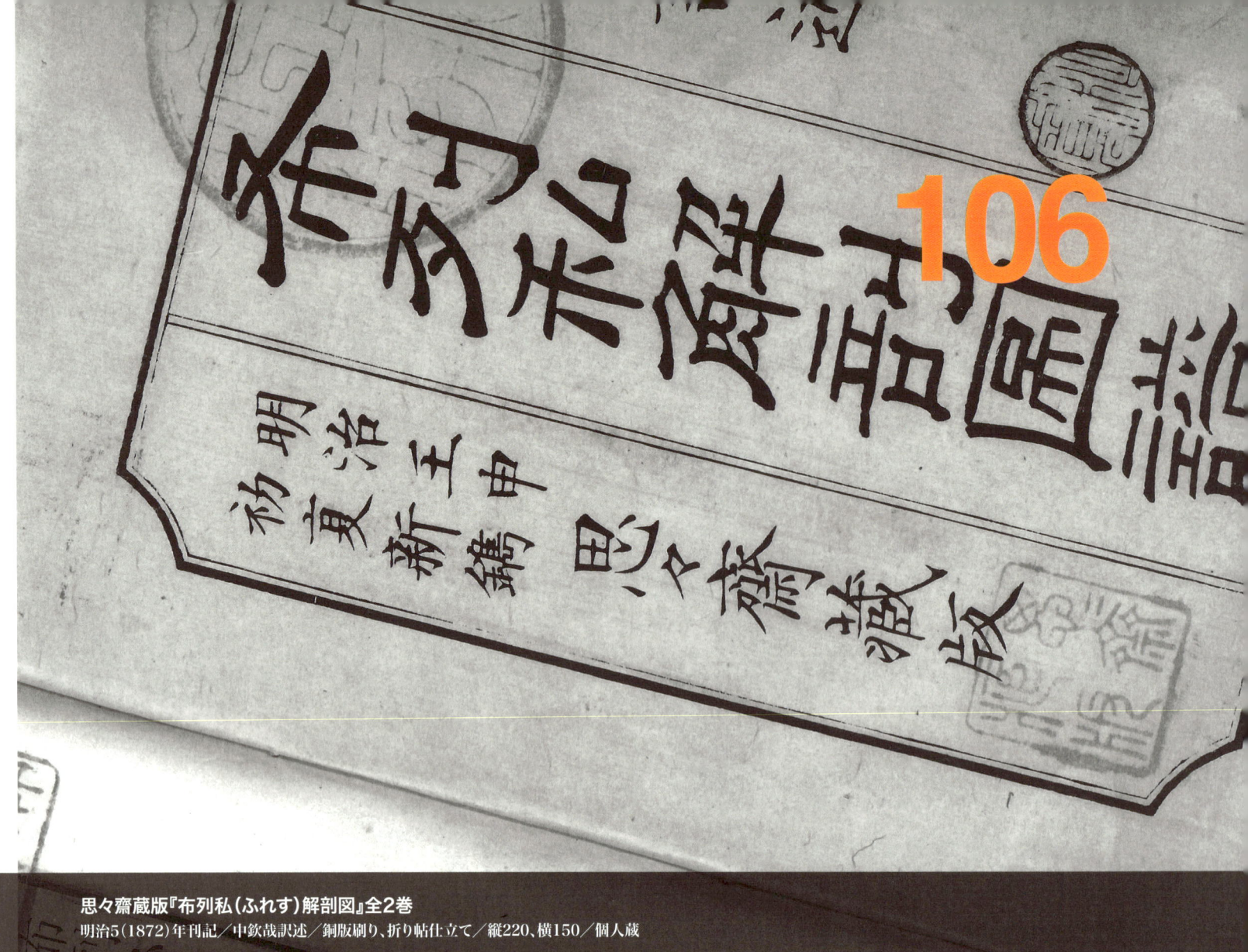

思々齋蔵版『布列私(ふれす)解剖図』全2巻
明治5(1872)年刊記／中欽哉訳述／銅版刷り、折り帖仕立て／縦220、横150／個人蔵

大坂鎮台病院の医師で、「欽哉」こと中定勝(1840-1903)が、ユトレヒト大学解剖学教授フレスの解剖学書第二版を翻訳したもの。解剖学的部位の名称を機械的に列挙した1冊と、それに連動した附図からなる。思々齋塾は、蘭学者中天游(1783-1835)が創始した私塾として知られる。

Fles' Anatomical Chart in Two Volumes, Shishisai Version
Published in 1872 / Translated by Kinya Naka / Copperplate printing, accordion binding / L220, W150 / Private collection

A translation by Sadakatsu (alias Kinya) Naka (1840 – 1903), physician at the Osaka garrison hospital, of the second edition of the anatomical reference book authored by Fles, professor of Anatomy at the University of Utrecht. It consists of a volume mechanically listing each anatomical part, and of associated illustrations. The Shishisai School was a private school established by Dutch-style scholar Tenyu Naka (1783 – 1835).

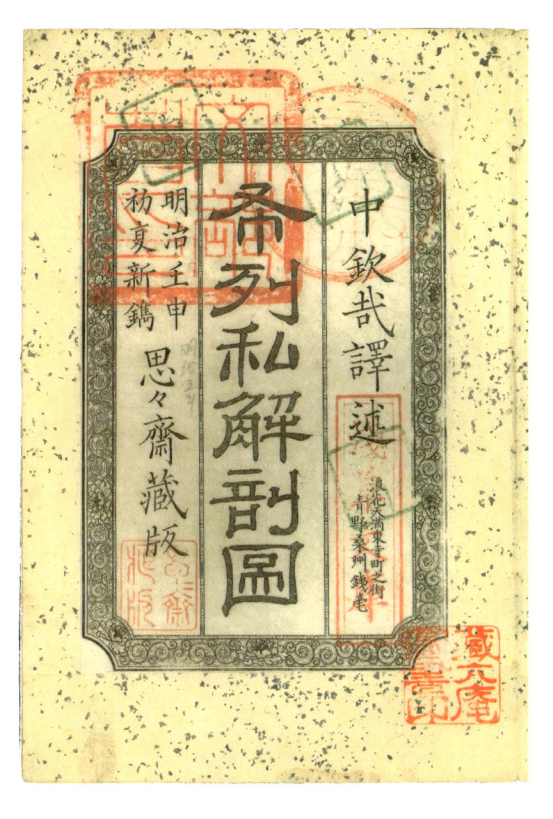

布列私解剖圖譜 完

希列私解剖圖
中欽武譯述
明治壬申初夏新鐫
思々齋藏版

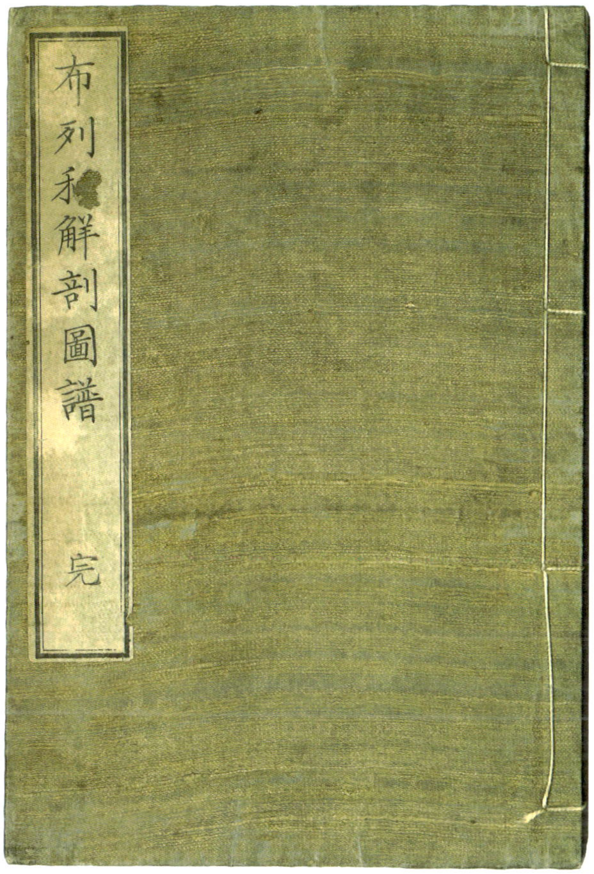

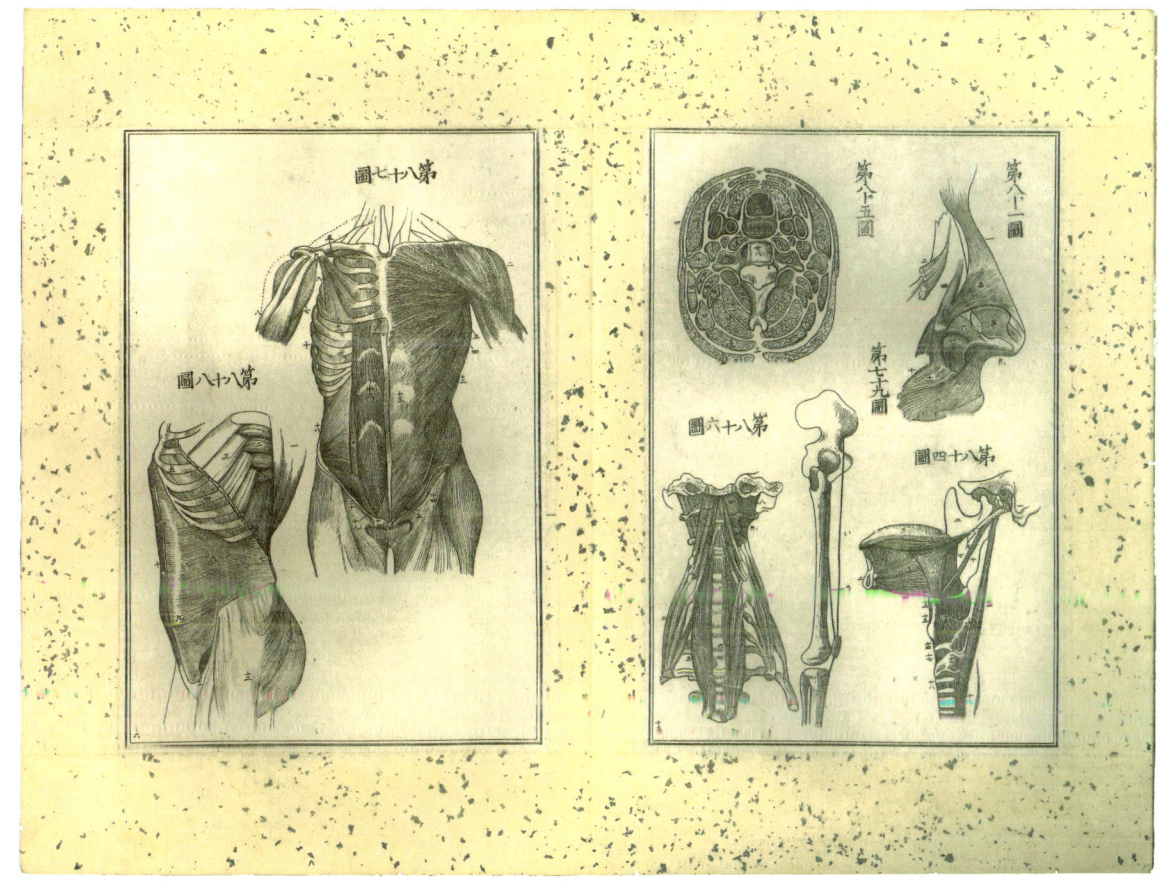

第八十七圖
第八十八圖
第八十一圖
第八十五圖
第七十九圖
第八十六圖
第八十四圖

108

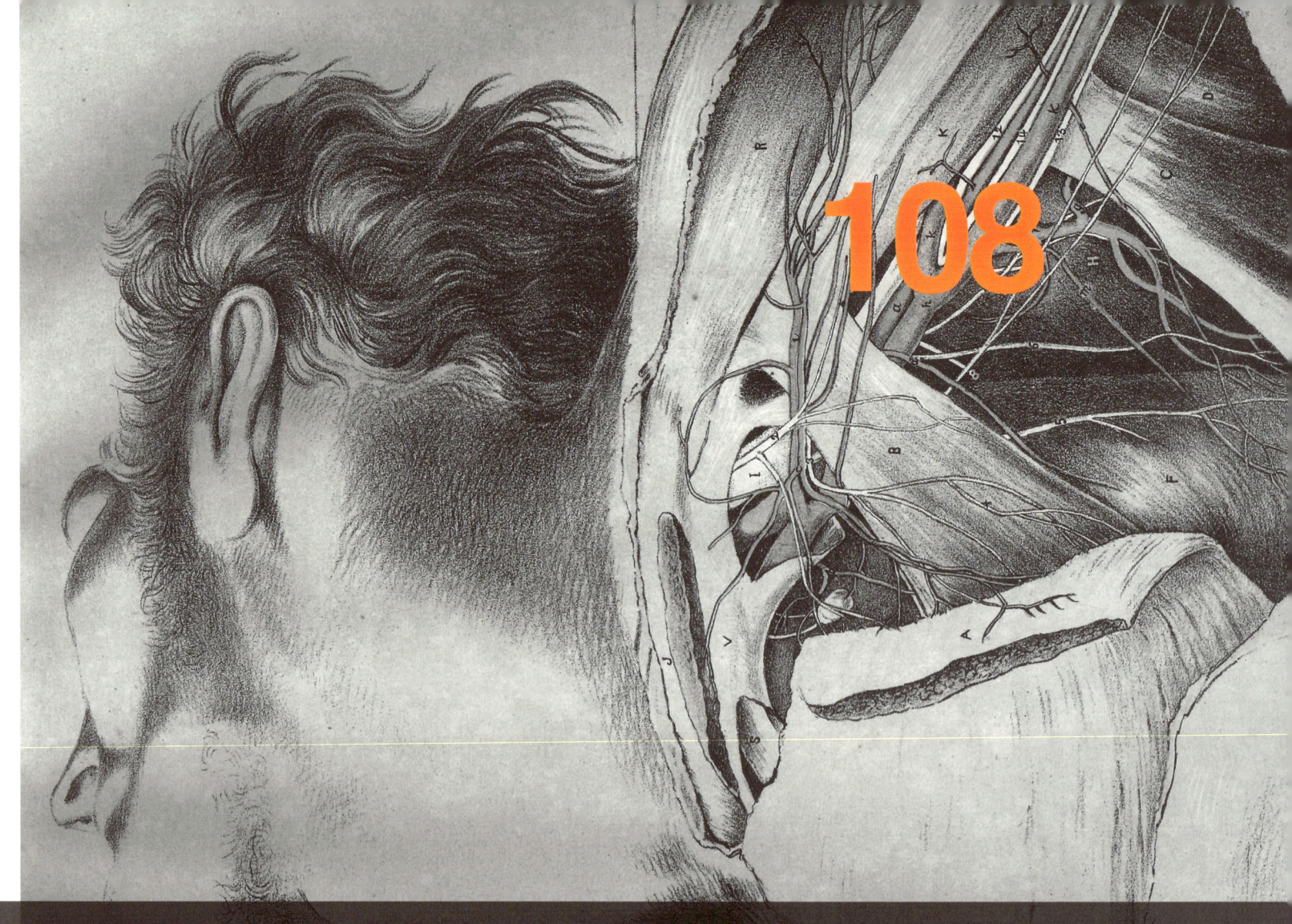

成医学校蔵版『人体局所解剖図』全58図付「和英対照表」
明治23（1890）年刊記／制作者未詳／多色石版、原装未詳／縦400、横285／個人蔵

石版の多色刷り印刷による国内で最初の解剖図譜である。底本とされたのは、ロンドンのユニヴァーシティ・カッレジで、1850年から解剖学教室を率いていたジョージ・ヴァイナー・エリス（1812–1900）が1867年にロンドンの書肆ジェームズ・ウォルトンからフォリオ判で出版した多色石版刷り『人体解剖図譜』である。原画を描き、石版に起こしたのは、南アフリカ出身の画工ジョージ・ヘンリー・フォード（1809–1876）である。動物画工として知られていたフォードは、1837年英国に渡り、当時は大英博物館で画工として働いていた。ロンドンのチャリング・クロスに近いニューポート・コートに工場を構えていたミンターン兄弟は、『ハチドリ科鳥類図譜』全2巻（1849／1861年）をはじめとする、剥製師ジョン・グールド（1804–1881）の鳥類図譜の印刷業者としても知られる。本図譜には各部の名称について、英語と日本語の対訳表を纏めた冊子が附されている。成医学校は現在の東京慈恵会医科大学の前身である。

Japanese-English Correspondence Chart Attached to the 58 Illustrations of the *Local Anatomical Drawings of the Human Body*, Seii Medical School Version
Published in 1890 / Author unknown / Polychrome lithography, original binding unknown / L400, W285 / Private collection

The first illustrated anatomical reference book to be printed in polychrome lithography in Japan. It is based on the polychrome lithography-printed *Dissection of the Human Body*, a book authored by George Viner Ellis (1812 – 1900), who taught anatomy at London's University College from 1850 on, and published in folio in 1867 by James Walton. It is the South African illustrator George Henry Ford (1809 – 1876) who drew the original illustrations and lithographed them. Ford, who is known as an animal illustrator, went to England in 1837, and worked as an illustrator at the British Museum. The Mintern brothers, whose factory was located in Newport Court near Charing Cross in London, are known for printing the ornithological illustrations of taxidermist John Gould (1804 – 1881), starting with the two volumes of *A Monograph of the Trochilidae or Humming Birds* (1849 / 1861). In this album, a booklet with a chart indicating the correspondences between English and Japanese for the denomination of each part is included. The Seii Medical School is the predecessor to the actual Jikei University.

第拾八圖

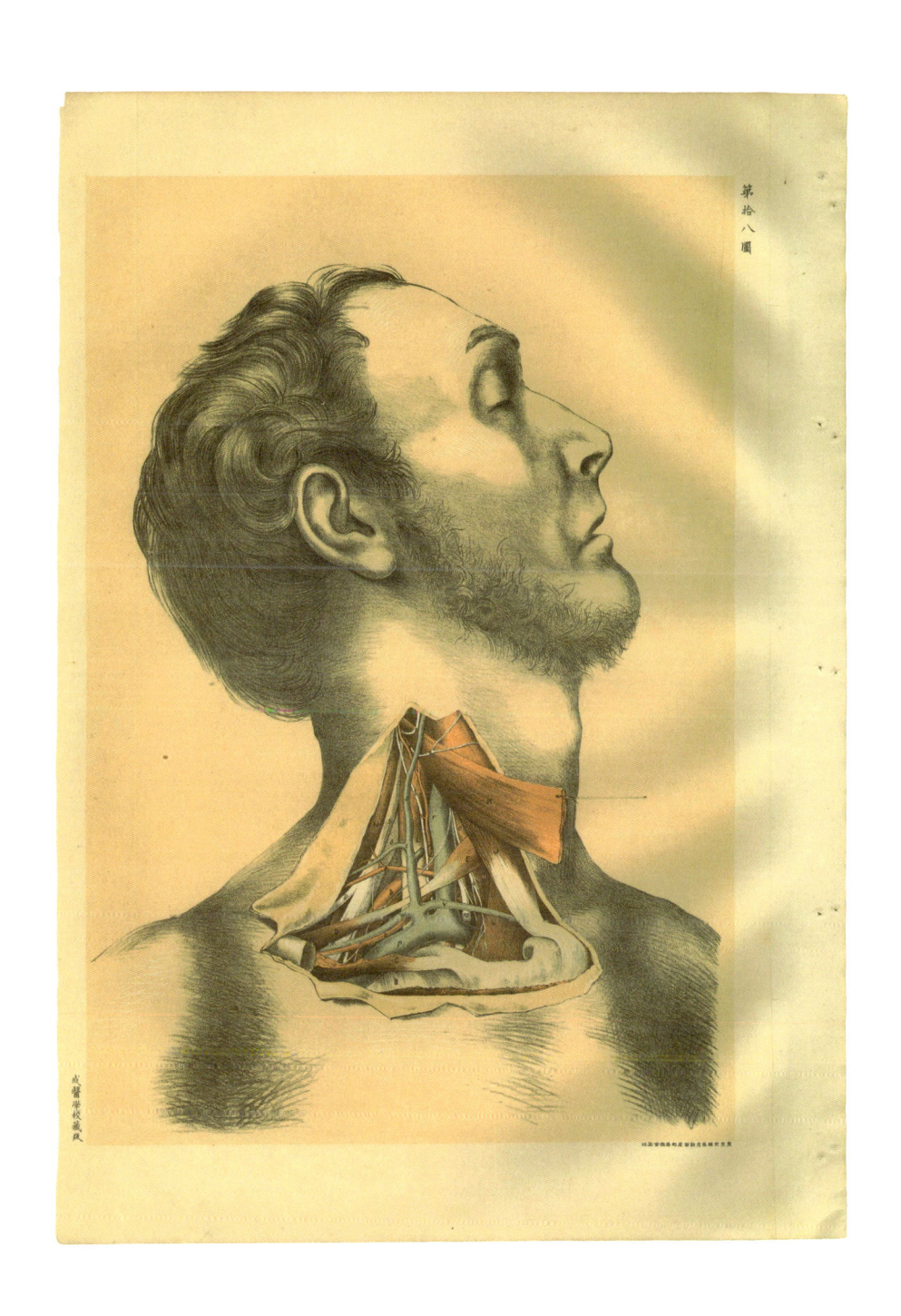

The Dawn of Modern Medicine in Japan: From Dutch Medicine to German Medical Science

Supervision: Exhibition Organization Committee for *The Dawn of Modern Medicine in Japan*
Design: Yoshiaki Nishino + Hiroyuki Sekioka
Photography: Norihiro Ueno + The University Museum, the University of Tokyo (UMUT)
Date of Publication: March 18, 2014
Publication: The University Museum, the University of Tokyo (UMUT)
Distribution: The University of Tokyo Press
Printing: Akita Kappan Printing
© Intermediatheque (IMT)
ISBN978-4-13-063403-8 Printed in Japan